# Homelessness, health care and welfare provision

Edited by Kevin Fisher and
John Collins

Foreword by David Widgery

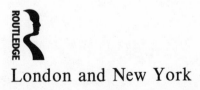

London and New York

First published in 1993
by Routledge
11 New Fetter Lane, London EC4P 4EE

Simultaneously published in the USA and Canada
by Routledge
29 West 35th Street, New York, NY 10001

Typeset in Times by Witwell Ltd, Southport
Printed and bound in Great Britain by
TJ Press (Padstow) Ltd, Padstow, Cornwall

*British Library Cataloguing in Publication Data*
A catalogue record for this book is available from the British Library.

*Library of Congress Cataloging in Publication Data*
Homelessness, health care, and welfare provision / edited by Kevin
  Fisher and John Collins ; foreword by David Widgery
  p.  cm.
  Includes bibliographical references and index.
  1. Homeless persons–Medical care–Great Britain. 2. Homeless
  persons–Medical care–United States. 3. Homeless persons–Services
  for–Great Britain. 4. Homeless persons–Services for–United
  States. I. Fisher, Kevin (Kevin John), 1958-  . II. Collins,
  John (John William), 1955-
  RA564.6.H63H65   1993
  362.1'0425–dc20                                        92-40458
                                                         CIP

ISBN 0-415-04999-7
    0-415-05000-6 (pbk)

# Contents

# Figures and tables

# Contributors

**John Balazs** is a General Practitioner in South London. Formerly a HHELP GP (1987–90).

**Elizabeth Bayliss** is Manager of the Community Psychiatry Research Unit, Hackney Hospital, London.

**Ian Boulton** is a Co-ordinator at No Fixed Abode: a co-ordinating service for voluntary agencies working with homeless people in the East End.

**John Collins** is a General Practitioner in Wapping, London. Formerly a HHELP GP (1985–87), he is presently GP Co-ordinator at HHELP.

**Jane Everton** is Area Manager of the Housing Corporation, London North West.

**Kevin Fisher** is a Probation Officer at the Middlesex Area Probation Service. Formerly a HHELP Social Worker (1987–89).

**Lynda Freimanis** is the Outreach Team Leader at the Drink Crisis Centre, London.

**David James** is a Senior Lecturer in Social Science at the University of Hertfordshire.

**Jim Reuler** is Chief of the Section of General Medicine at the Veterans' Affairs Medical Centre, and Professor of Medicine at Oregon Health Sciences University, Portland, Oregon.

**Philip Timms** is a Senior Lecturer in the Mental Health Team for Single Homeless People.

# Foreword

*David Widgery*

Government ministers fulminate about falling moral standards and magistrates bemoan the plague of able-bodied beggars infesting the West End. Welfare managers boast about their 'efficiency' savings and buck-passing schemes for 'internal markets', while the working-class poor lack fresh food, sound education and clean air. East End doctors report that housing 'is the most difficult social problem of the day . . . that the very class of persons most urgently requiring some better accommodation is the class for which the large building trusts will not supply'. And a senior officer of the Salvation Army elaborates 'there is a depth below that of the dweller in the slums. It is that of the dweller in the street, who has not even a lair in the slums which they can call their own.'

*Plus ça change* indeed. Tower Hamlets of a hundred years ago and the words of Dr Joseph Loane, Medical Officer of Health for the Whitechapel District and General Booth have a familiar ring to those of us who work in the East End's health service today. Now as then, deepening cycles of economic recession bite harshly into the fragile domestic finances of the poor. Now as then, government policy of *laissez faire* economics, public service cuts and less eligible welfare combine to lever those most in need of mainstream care to the mercies of the charitable and voluntary sector. Now as then, it is the homeless who experience poverty in its most extreme form and although they need more health care, they get the least, often of the wrong kind. Too often the 'No-Fixed-Abodes' are treated as human bric-à-brac whose fits, fractures and swollen feet are somehow less entitled to proper treatment. The names that ought to be remembered after reading this book are the politicians, bankers and developers who are guilty not merely of failing to deal with the problem of homelessness but, in reality, of fuelling it. We should also never forget people like Alan from Tower Hamlets Mission, Thomas Frazer in Hackney and Arthur

Stevens in South London who died in pain and unattended, died of homelessness, chucked out of 'accident and emergency', spurned in doorways, unexamined by so-called doctors, tut-tutted about but not aided by society.

Homelessness *is* the big issue. And the bad old days are here again. During the slump of the 1930s, George Orwell noted, in 1933 when the national government had slashed the value of benefits and introduced the Means Test, that his down and out fellow-travellers were 'of all kinds and ages . . . some hardened tramps . . . some factory hands out of work . . . a clerk . . . two certainly imbeciles'. The contemporary homeless are still more varied. They are not just the single men with a taste for strong lager, the demented evicted from the asylums which at least kept them warm or the jobless forced to travel in search of work by the industrial clearance of the North East, Scotland and South Wales. They are re-possessed mortgagees from the once prosperous South East, teenagers 'in care' fleeing institutions which have failed and sometimes abused them, teenagers who have been thrown out by parents or step-parents, ex-children, maybe yours or mine, who have committed the crime of growing up and who simply want a place of their own even if it is an insecure squat. And behind them mass an uncounted multitude – families who endure gross overcrowding in unmaintained 'hard-to-let' council property or unsuitable hotels, those in work or at college who are obliged to turn over most of their income to rack-renting landlords, people who sleep on a rota of front-room sofas, the refugees and asylum seekers whose papers are being processed, the families evicted from their rightful council accommodation because they visited their country of origin for too long – all people who may have addresses but certainly don't have homes. These homeless people aren't suffering from some mysterious character defect, rather they are the human consequences of the neo-liberal economics dominant in Britain since the mid-1970s which has now catastrophically failed even on its own terms. But which was utilized as a pretext for national government to opt out conveniently of any political responsibility for public housing. What a change from Harold Macmillan's proud boast of over 300,000 new dwellings completed in 1953 to the situation where, according to the building employers, over 580 jobs, ranging from architects to roofing apprentices, have been lost in the industry *each day* between 1989 and 1992.

If, and the likelihood is remote, the direction of policy were reversed tomorrow the backlog of neglect would take years to repair. Health workers can't be expected to substitute for the fundamental change of direction required. But, in East London, stemming from the pioneering work of Barbara Burke-Masters and with the help of some officials from the DSS and the Family Heath Services, the HHELP team has made real progress in improving the lamentable standards of health care provided by the NHS to the homeless. Like-minded workers in Central and South London have sought to do the same. There is perhaps not such a long way between William Booth's pony, trap and two nurses and the black cab used by the Drink Crisis Centre to ferry their clients to better medical care. But, the modern pioneers have been innovative in their use of specialist, on-site services to integrate and propel the homeless towards the mainstream of NHS primary care, they have successfully used multidisciplinary teamwork and they have educated, trained and arranged finances to enable fellow practitioners in the East End to provide high-quality health care for the homeless. Their findings should be on the desk of every urban GP, in the staff room of every accident and emergency department and on the bedside table of every comfortable politician who has passed the buck on this issue.

# Acknowledgements

Many people have contributed, directly or indirectly, to the work which led to the production of this book. The editors have worked in primary care services for single homeless people in the East End of London since 1985 and would like to thank all of our past and present patients/clients for teaching us much of what we know.

Specific thanks are due to the late Hugh Jones, formerly in the finance section of the then DHSS. His enthusiasm and efforts enabled the funding of the original East London Homeless Health Care Team (HHELP), which brought us together as social worker and salaried general practitioner.

We would also like to thank all past and present HHELP team members for their work and support; all local voluntary sector agencies and staff upon whom this work depends; the HHELP management committee members and Mr Alan Bennett, General Manager of City and East London Family Health Services Authority, for his imaginative management input into the HHELP team since its inception and his present continuing interest in our work.

Thanks also are due to Maureen Shaw for her repeated typing of miles of manuscript and to Gill Weedon for transcribing many hours of taped interviews. Alison Wooldridge and Ewen Rose each read parts of the manuscript and we are grateful for their helpful comments. Heather Gibson, our editor at Routledge, has provided continuous encouragement and unfailingly tolerated our shortcomings as authors.

Lastly we would like to thank our partners, Claire Fisher and Shenda Collins, for putting up with our presences and absences over the last two years, and for their unwavering support.

## POSTSCRIPT

We would especially like to thank Dr David Widgery who contributed the Foreword to this book only a few weeks before his sudden death on 26 October 1992.

David was a leading light in East End General Practice for 20 years and an inspiration to many local health professionals and students. He was also well known as an author, journalist, activist and political historian.

David will be remembered as an informed and radical thinker in all these spheres but we especially remember him for his concern for homeless people, his personal contribution to their care and for his encouragement and support of our work.

# Introduction

*Kevin Fisher and John Collins*

Being homeless is rotten. In a world of statistics and social analysis this is sometimes overlooked. . . . For a start you aren't needed by anyone. . . . You have nowhere to go and nothing to do except get through the day and night. You wander amidst bustling crowds of clean, well fed and busy people. . . . You have little money, no friends and almost no content to your life save to keep warm in libraries or queue up for your benefit at the social security. Worst of all you are alone and that brings with it an increasing sense of isolation.

(Cox and Cox 1977)

In recent years the problem of homelessness has escalated into a critical social issue, stimulating a wave of concern from the voluntary sector, pressure groups and, occasionally, policy makers. This concern has been provoked by the seeming upsurge in the numbers of homeless people sleeping on the streets of our cities. As shopfronts, underpasses and doorways were transformed into hotels for the needy the shock of homelessness became public. And homelessness, as Marcuse has observed, is shocking.

It is immediately shocking to the homeless, but ultimately to the system that produces homelessness. Homelessness is shocking to those who are not homeless because it exposes misery in the midst of plenty, and represents alienation from home in a home-based society.

(Marcuse 1988: 68)

Public awareness of the problem of homelessness was not heightened only by the escalation of the problem, nor by the attendant media coverage. Rather there was a gradual realization that people who were homeless were not all 'lazy crazy drunks' but people like us: women and children, men with trades and young people with hopes and aspirations; individuals with simply nowhere to sleep.

While this heightened awareness of the problem of single homelessness has been slow to filter through to certain policy-making forums, public service providers and some sections of the media, it is acknowledged by those agencies working with the homeless. One of the first indications of changing attitudes was a changing language; it was no longer acceptable to call homeless people vagrants, outcasts, tramps or dossers. The voluntary sector was able to see at firsthand that homelessness was a problem affecting people from all social classes, backgrounds and cultures. As conceptions of homelessness were 'normalized', voluntary agencies began to attempt to access mainstream services on behalf of the men and women who used their centres. Unfortunately, many organizations found that mainstream providers did not see single homeless people as being entitled to use their services. Local authority housing departments were reluctant to place anyone single and homeless on their waiting lists, even when they were evidently vulnerable. Social services seemed to view single homelessness as being the responsibility of the voluntary sector, health care for homeless people is often poor and fragmented and general practitioners are often reluctant to register homeless people on anything but a temporary basis.

The problems faced by single homeless people in gaining access to good quality health care have until recently proved to be particularly intractable. This state of affairs may seem to be at odds with one of the fundamental principles of the National Health Service; namely, equal access for all. The Black Report (1980) showed, however, that, for disadvantaged groups in society, it is extremely difficult to exercise this right. Poverty, unemployment and homelessness are not conducive to good health. The pressures they impose can make health a very low priority, and the vulnerability homeless people feel makes the bureaucracy associated with medical practice seem threatening: one reason why many homeless people, particularly those sleeping rough, do not register with GPs.

The discriminatory treatment of some single homeless men and women by the health service is evidenced by the following reports which were collected by the Medical Campaign Project.

Mr K, homeless and aged 54, had an attack of pain in his chest and arm and was breathless and fainting. He was taken to a nearby hospital, by workers from Arlington Drop-in Centre, in a semi-conscious state. The duty doctor only queried whether he had been drinking. Mr K does not drink, but the doctor kept asking him how much he had drunk. After 12 minutes the doctor said that Mr K had nothing wrong and that he could go. The worker explained that Mr K could not even walk. After another examination Mr K was found to have blood clots. He had to have major heart surgery and spent six months in hospital and convalescent homes. He has made a good recovery. If Mr K had gone to the hospital on his own he would probably be dead today.

Seventy-seven-year-old Alan was found by workers from the Tower Hamlets Mission. He had been sleeping rough and looked ill. Police and ambulance men refused to take him to hospital dismissing him as drunk. Eventually the workers took him to the London Hospital where his foot was found to be badly infected. After reluctantly admitting him in casualty, doctors discovered that he had been admitted two months before to have a toe amputated, had been discharged and that the wound had become infected. He died of renal failure two days after being re-admitted.

The source of this reluctance by health professionals to engage with homeless men and women lies in a stereotyped view of homelessness in which individual inadequacy, social pathology and deviance have been the dominant themes. Indeed, it is evident that one of the most impenetrable barriers to access to high quality health care has been, and remains, the portrayal of homeless people as being largely irredeemable and therefore a potential waste of time and resources. In essence, like other marginalized sections of society, homeless people have been labelled as bad, mad or sad; criminal, insane or alcoholic.

Legislation, the dominant mechanism of social control, has been variously used over the centuries to retain a modicum of control over homeless people. Significantly it has reflected the interests of status groups in society. Thus the vagrancy statutes in the Middle Ages sanctioned the landowners' need for cheap labour and obviated the need to compete for a scarce resource. From the sixteenth century onwards the focal concern changed as the vagrancy statutes reflected the new commercial spirit of the age and the concern of the authorities to protect mercantile interests. The nineteenth century also witnessed a profound change in attitudes. Homelessness continued to be surrounded by spectres of deviancy; indeed, one writer described the homeless deviant as 'the chrysalis of every species of criminal' (Friedman 1886 cited by Steele 1979). Perhaps the dominant theme is of the homeless person as a social evil, a totally immoral entity who would infect the more deserving poor. This Victorian inheritance can be seen in the continuing existence of the casual wards now euphemistically called resettlement units and in the archaic vagrancy laws. The persistence of these reflects society's perception of a continuing need to control some of its suspicious or undesirable members.

The conceptualization of the homeless as mad also has a long history but a more recent prominence. Grey (1931), for example, noted that 'A very large proportion of boys upon the road are mentally peculiar, indeed if they were not, they would not be on the road.' Whitley (1955) drew similar conclusions. 'To his environment the down and out contributes nothing. To exist in it he must be as psychopathic as his neighbour.'

Snow *et al.* suggest that what they term the 'myth of pervasive mental illness' among the homeless is the result of 'the medicalisation of the problem of homelessness, a misplaced emphasis on the causal role of de-institutionalisation and the heightened visibility of homeless individuals who are mentally ill' (Snow *et al.* 1986).

The medicalisation of or, more accurately, the treatment approach to homelessness has been prompted by the fields of both psychology and psychiatry. Early attempts to identify the homeless personality are epitomized in the work of Boris Levinson. In 'The homeless man: a psychological enigma', Levinson argued that by looking at the homeless

as cultural deviants or mutants, and as the end result of a moral, social and familial crisis we can no longer consider them as being in the thralldom of a disease process, these men are by-products of our culture; they have gone through aversive learning experiences which we have provided for them. In a sense we can see the dilemma of the modern world in the homeless man. In stark light, in majestic simplicity, we can see what happens to a man when society does not offer him the opportunity of posing or pondering the question 'Who am I?' 'Where am I going?' 'What is the meaning of it all?'

(Levinson 1963: 592)

In the same article Levinson explored the unconscious psychodynamics of homelessness and argued that a common feature of the homeless psyche is a poor psychosexual history resulting from a turbulent relationship with the mother figure. Levinson's basic hypothesis was that the homeless man, having been rejected by 'significant others', descends into the homeless milieu; in so doing he chooses, subconsciously, to withdraw from life in order to enjoy the freedom of the homeless existence.

While Levinson's reasoning and language may at times sound

faintly ridiculous, his work remains influential. Homelessness as a chosen lifestyle is a concept still bandied about by policy makers.

David Willets, for instance, formerly a member of Mrs Thatcher's policy unit, used the concept of the 'chosen lifestyle' to reduce homelessness to a bizarre expression of New Right ideology when he argued that the increasing numbers of men and women sleeping on the streets were 'an example of a rise in individualism and taste for independence' (*Independent* 24 October 1989).

A further by-product of the Levinson-type thesis is the argument that 'while it may be possible to get the homeless off skid row it is impossible to get skid row out of the homeless'. Levinson gives this myth credibility with his theory of homelessness as a learned behaviour. This myth has often been propagated by the wardens of dubious hostels which the homeless eschew in favour of the streets. With no prospect of permanent accommodation the street is often cleaner and safer than the hostel.

Nevertheless, notions of rehabilitation predominate, particularly in some sections of voluntary sector, and, while the rationale varies, getting skid row out of the man generally underpins much of their work. There is no question that many of the homeless have poor social skills and low levels of confidence. However, lack of access to permanent accommodation and unemployment remain their primary handicaps. No amount of treatment or rehabilitation will do anything to alleviate these.

The psychopathological approach views homelessness as primarily resulting from a disease-based entity. There is little doubt that many homeless men and women suffer from psycho-social stress as a result of their lack of a home or job. Furthermore, it is evident that a minority of the homeless are the victims of various acute and chronic forms of mental illness. This is clearly demonstrated in the empirical data in later chapters. Central to the argument here is the proposition that conceptualizations of the homeless as mad have been abetted by political, personal and ideological self-interest. As Ropers has noted:

When claims of some segments of the mental health profession regarding the prevalence of mental illness are examined these claims often appear to be scientifically vacuous. If the contentions that homelessness is caused by de-institutionalisation or that homelessness is itself a symptom of mental illness, and that nearly half or more of the homeless are mentally ill, can be demonstrated not to be supported by scientific evidence then perhaps such assertions are ideological in nature.

(Ropers 1988: 167)

An important proponent of the idea of the homeless as mentally ill is the American psychiatrist Dr Ellen Basuk. Her article 'Is homelessness a mental health problem?' (Bassuk *et al.* 1984) was based on interviews with seventy-eight men, women and children in an emergency night-shelter in Boston, Massachusetts. The vast majority were found to have severe mental health problems: 91 per cent were given primary psychiatric diagnoses, 40 per cent had psychoses, 29 per cent were chronic alcoholics and 21 per cent had personality disorders. On the basis of this study Bassuk argued that deinstitutionalization had led to the institutions of homelessness, such as night-shelters, and the streets becoming open asylums.

The content and underlying thesis of this study have been contested and will again be disputed in later chapters. Here it serves as an example of how a no doubt well-meaning attempt by the psychiatric profession to colonize the homelessness problem can, with attendant media hype, influence and shape the public view. Such attempts, if successful, enable a complete redefinition of the problem. No longer is homelessness a housing problem or a failure of housing policy. It is a mental health problem and therefore a failure of mental health policy.

Snow *et al.*, in an article entitled 'On the precariousness of measuring insanity in insane contexts', point to the danger of misreading and therefore diagnosing the behaviour of homeless people as indicative of mental impairment when it can perhaps be explained as an adaptive behaviour. As Snow *et al.* note:

> the situations in which homeless people live constitute, in a very real sense, such insane contexts thus increasing the prospect that adaptation to them may be misread as insanity. So long as contextually adaptive behaviours are confused with truly symptomatic behaviours, assessments of the incidence of mental illness on the streets will be fraught with error and we suspect, skewed diagnosis.
>
> (Snow *et al.* 1988: 195)

Historical, psychological and psychopathological concepts of homelessness have all influenced public opinion, decision makers, service providers, social policy and ultimately definitions of homelessness. It is clear that such concepts play an important role in neutralizing the political implications of homelessness. This is illustrated in their impact on decision makers and legislators, particularly in relation to the formulation of statutory definitions. Definitions can, when accurately constructed, give a clear insight into the nature and causes of homelessness. Alternatively, they are a convenient tool for limiting access to resources.

In spite of this panoply of ignorance, fear and stigmatization, health care services for single homeless people have been developed. In areas which have particularly large populations of single homeless people special projects have been set up to bridge the gap in service provision. One of the first of these was the East London Homeless Health Project (HHELP), which was set up in 1986 by the Secretary of State for Health as one of two three-year pilot projects to investigate the primary health care needs of single homeless people in London. The decision to set up HHELP largely resulted from publicity surrounding the work of Barbara Burke-Masters, a nursing sister. Supported by a local GP and working from an East End day centre, Sister Burke-Masters' work with the homeless drew media attention when her clinic was closed, in 1985, after she was threatened with legal action by the Pharmaceutical Society. This publicity, both supportive and critical, fuelled the debate on the paucity of local provision and actually moved the statutory authorities to action.

This book was conceived at a time when the HHELP project was facing an uncertain future. Its funding was coming to an end and the team's contracts were about to expire. Both team members and the voluntary agencies from which they operated feared that, with no funding in sight, the team's services to the single homeless could be entirely lost. As a result of intensive lobbying, and a not insignificant amount of media attention, funding was made available. Since 1989 HHELP has become a permanent part of the East End primary health and social care provision and a major part of its remit is to encourage the people it sees into mainstream and generic health and social services. The continued existence of HHELP and the creation of other special services nationally signify that there is a more widespread acceptance that homeless people have a right to health care and that addresslessness should not be a barrier to access. This notion of equality of access is a central theme, emphasized throughout the book.

In the opening chapter Jane Everton examines the impact of housing, social security and health policy on the problem of single homelessness. Definitions of homelessness are considered, as are attempts to gauge the number of people who are homeless at any one time. The chapter's main focus is on the effect of national and local housing policies on single people who are homeless in London. The vigorous promotion of owner-occupation together with the decline in the private rented sector have had the effect of limiting the housing choices of single people on low incomes. At the same time, the ability of local authority housing departments to house even small numbers of homeless single people has been limited by financial constraints and the priority need of homeless families. Changes in the financing of housing associations have also led to concerns about their ability to develop new housing schemes for the single homeless population. Access to permanent accommodation has been hindered, too, by the replacement of traditional direct access hostels with a range of smaller hostels rather than permanent housing, the belief being that supportive hostel provision was a necessary step for most single and homeless people. Access to both mainstream housing and hostel accommodation has also been hampered by changes in the social security system particularly affecting young people. Everton ends by opening up the debate concerning the most appropriate mechanism for ensuring that single and homeless men and women have access to adequate health care.

Issues concerning access are the subject of the following chapter in which Kevin Fisher and John Collins highlight the difficulties homeless ill people have encountered in accessing medical provision. As general practitioners are the traditional gatekeepers to health care services, a key issue is their willingness, or otherwise, to register men and women who are single and homeless. The problem of low registration rates, particularly among rough sleepers is not simply a question of GP refusal. Fisher and Collins attempt to explain why many people who are using insecure accommodation or sleeping rough are reluctant to use primary health care services, significant factors being previous experience of stigmatization and low health expectations. The chapter moves on to examine the way in which homeless people use emergency and secondary services and concludes with an exploration of the effects of the 1991 NHS reforms.

In Chapter 3 John Balazs uses data gathered by the East London Homeless Health Care Team to describe and analyse the health problems experienced by the single homeless population. Wherever possible, comparisons are made and contrasts are drawn with the housed population in order to be able to demonstrate the impact that homelessness has on individual well-being. Balazs highlights the fact that homelessness is a precursor to higher rates of certain types of morbidity and, conversely, that health problems may cause homelessness. The chapter opens with a comprehensive profile of the people who have used the HHELP's services and moves on to a detailed discussion of the health care problems they presented. In doing this Balazs differentiates between different sub-groups within the homeless population in order to demonstrate that their experience of ill-health is not a homogeneous one. The chapter concludes with the observation that access to both affordable accommodation and high quality health care is a prerequisite to any improvement in the health status of the thousands of men and women who are literally 'out in the cold'.

The plight of homeless people with mental health problems has in recent years created an upsurge in public debate concerning the fate of patients discharged from psychiatric hospitals. In Chapter 4 Philip Timms traces the roots of this concern and discusses the causal factors relating to rising numbers of homeless people with mental health problems. As well as describing some of the innovative projects that have developed both in Britain and the United States, the chapter looks at how mainstream psychiatry could provide a more responsive and flexible service for homeless people.

The needs of homeless street drinkers have largely been ignored by society because they represent the stereotypical homeless person. In Chapter 5 Linda Freimanis outlines the development of the Drink Crisis Centre outreach team which works with homeless street drinkers. The team have developed a model of intervention which is both immediate and accessible. A key feature of this outreach team's work is that it operates in conjunction with a number of other agencies in the field rather than in traditional isolation. The chapter also describes how a multidisciplinary approach has facilitated a number of developments such as 'holding beds' and 'joint care planning'.

In the following chapter Ian Boulton describes some of the particular problems encountered by young homeless people. Young people become homeless for a number of reasons ranging from overcrowding at home to child abuse. Once homeless they face a punitive benefits system, a drastic shortage of accessible accommodation and exploitative elders. Boulton describes how young people can be particularly vulnerable to ill health, often because they simply don't know where to get help. The chapter concludes by arguing that only a strategy which emphasizes statutory responsibility will eradicate the problem.

A number of mechanisms for delivering health care to single homeless people have been developed. In Chapter 7 Elizabeth Bayliss identifies three models of health care provision: namely, separate schemes, special schemes and fully integrated services. Bayliss highlights the advantages and disadvantages of each model and particular consideration is given to factors such as access, the range of treatment offered, their ability to change the homeless person's immediate environment and finally each model's ability to meet the differing needs within the homeless population. The chapter concludes by listing a number of recommendations for action.

In Chapter 8 David James looks at the development of campaigning on issues relating to health care and single homelessness. Until the establishment of the Medical Campaign project in 1986 issues relating to poor health and homelessness had mainly been highlighted by locally based community health councils and voluntary agencies, generally in response to allegations of mistreatment and malpractice. The chapter highlights the fact that the homeless field is itself divided over the most appropriate mechanisms for delivering adequate health care to the homeless population. Recognizing that this is partly due to the heterogeneity of the homelessness problem, James advocates the building of coalitions between homeless people and specific interest groups in order to develop a campaigning platform.

In the final chapter Jim Reuler describes how a number of health care programmes have been established in the United States in order to provide medical and social care to the homeless. This chapter illustrates how a health care system based on private insurance fails to care for the medically indigent despite the provision of public health insurance programmes, public hospitals and a specific health care programme for veterans. Professor Reuler describes how special projects, some based on the outreach principle, others in centralized clinics, have been developed around the United States in order to plug the gaps in health care delivery. One of the largest of these, the Johnson-Pew Programme, allocated funds for research into the health care problems of the homeless and their main findings highlight how common afflictions combined with a chaotic and marginal lifestyle can evolve into chronic health problems. Special programmes have played a significant role in enabling the US homeless to gain access to appropriate health care. However, as Professor Reuler observes, without adequate housing and a universal health care system, such developments will remain a 'band aid' solution to a health care disaster.

This book was written because the editors' experience led them to believe that historical perceptions of single homeless people and their health care needs were outmoded. We argue that homelessness excludes its victims from statutory health care provision, that the health status of homeless people is more closely related to inadequate housing than to individual pathology or the inaccessibility of health care and that social policy effectively determines the extent, demography and epidemiology of homelessness. Further, we wished to demonstrate that there have been a number of significant developments in the provision of health care to single homeless people in recent years.

Most of the contributors to this book currently work with homeless people and have been responsible for the development of some of the innovative and creative services which are described.

The authors' different perspectives have developed from their individual experience and knowledge of homeless people. Their contributions illustrate our argument from these different viewpoints and demonstrate the underlying day to day struggle that those working with homeless people go through in trying to resolve the problems of meeting complex health needs in a context of limited resources and inadequate housing provision.

It is perhaps inevitable that in any novel and dynamic area of health care or welfare provision, service providers will have different opinions about the most effective methods of intervention. Health care for homeless people is no exception, particularly given its multi-disciplinary base. Such differences are reflected in several of the following chapters and it is hoped that the opinions expressed by their authors will serve to widen and inform debate.

## REFERENCES

Bassuk, E., Rubin, L. and Lauriat, A. (1984) 'Is homelessness a mental health problem?', *The American Journal of Psychiatry*, 141 (12): 1546–50.

Cox, A. and Cox, G. (1977) *Building a Partial View of Detached Work with Homeless Young People*, London: National Youth Bureau.

Grey, F. (1931) *The Tramp: His Meaning and Being*, London: Dent.

Levinson, B. (1963) 'The homeless man: a psychological enigma', *Mental Hygiene*, 47: 596–9.

Marcuse, P. (1988) 'Neutralizing homelessness', *Socialist Review*, 18 (1): 69–96.

Ropers, R.H. (1988) *The Invisible Homeless: a New Urban Ecology*, New York: Insight Books.

Snow, D.A., Baker, S.G., Anderson, L. and Martin, M. (1986) 'The myth of pervasive mental illness among the homeless', *Social Problems*, 33 (5): 407–22.

Snow, D.A., Baker, S.G. and Anderson L. (1988) 'On the precariousness of measuring insanity in insane contexts', *Social Problems*, 35 (2): 192–6.

Steele, D.W. (1979) 'Vagrancy – social origins and response', *FARE Study Paper No 1*, Federation of Alcoholic Rehabilitation Establishments.

Watson, S. and Austenberry, H. (1986) *Housing and Homelessness: a Feminist Perspective*, London: Routledge & Kegan Paul.

Whitley, J.S. (1955) 'Down and out in London: mental illness in the lower social groups', *Lancet* 2: 608–10.

Willets, D. (1989) 'Sleeping rough is a chosen lifestyle' *Independent* 24 October.

# 1 Single homelessness and social policy

*Jane Everton*

## INTRODUCTION

Finding a clear, simple definition of single homelessness has always been problematic. The label 'homeless family' immediately brings to mind the plight of children with no secure home, and their needs are quickly established. For people who are single and homeless there are no such easy labels to define their need. Either they are grouped into particular areas of need such as the young, alcohol abusers, people with AIDS/HIV or people who are mentally ill, or a specific image of single homeless people is put forward, the much over-used picture of the old man on the streets with bottle in hand still being the most common.

Professionally, too, definitions of single homelessness have lapsed into simple labels. The term 'special needs' is used to cover everyone from the person who is simply single and without a home to someone who is severely mentally ill and requiring considerable support and expert care. It is possible that such labels and easy definitions do not count for much, that what matters is developing housing for people in need. However, labels can be powerful, particularly in combination with evocative images of people sleeping on the streets. Inevitably they influence public understanding of single homelessness and the way in which arguments are made for the housing and care solutions needed to meet the problem. In this chapter, the developing understanding of and changing response to single homelessness in London will be explored. London is a useful example to take, not only because of the size of the problem there, but also because of the specific short-term and long-term programmes which have been developed.

## DEFINITIONS AND CONCEPTS

People who are single and homeless are most easily defined as who they are not, rather than as who they are. The main body of legislation affecting them remains the 1977 Housing (Homeless Persons) Act, now incorporated into the 1985 Housing Act. Despite a recent review of the legislation, most single homeless people are still excluded from statutory help from their local councils. Only if they are over pensionable age, mentally ill or vulnerable will they receive help. Young single women who are pregnant or are single mothers are also entitled to help. Often such assistance depends upon a council's definition of 'vulnerability', and on whether a person is deemed to have made themselves 'intentionally' homeless.

Consequently, single homeless people have been excluded from the main framework of housing services for people in need. Local authorities are encouraged to give guidance on other housing or advice resources in the area, but this help is often limited and varies considerably.

People become homeless and single for many reasons: family/relationship breakdown; insecure housing; loss of a job; or the simple lack of affordable housing. This is why it is so difficult to define 'single homelessness': labels attached to the problem often confuse other possible contributory causes of homelessness with that of simply having no home. For instance, young homeless people have been encouraged to return to the parental home as a solution to their homelessness. The problem therefore becomes one of rebellious youth, and not one of a young adult rightly seeking to set up home alone. Such confusion has also been evident in the professional approach to single homelessness. For example, homeless single people with alcohol problems can be expected not to drink when they are in a hostel, and, if they do, can lose their housing. It may be impossible for people to give up alcohol in this way, and the demand appears to put their housing needs in second place.

The range of needs amongst people who are single and homeless has led to a profusion of voluntary projects specializing in particular areas. Hostels for ex-offenders, young people leaving care, people with mental illness, women or elderly homeless people have been developed because of a lack of necessary support or appropriate provision for these people in general hostels. Such services are essential and have helped to develop an understanding that for many people good housing and services are equally important. However, this focus on specific areas of housing need has also reinforced the idea that a label additional to homelessness is necessary in order to establish need and gain funding and support.

Changes to hostel provision in London over the past ten years also reflect a change in general definitions of single homelessness. In the early 1980s, the closure of large hostels, such as the DHSS-owned Camberwell Resettlement Unit or 'Spike', and the proposed closure of three Rowton hostels encouraged the idea that homeless people needed some form of small hostel provision where support could be given before moving into permanent housing. While this may have been true for many of the men in Camberwell, it is not the case for all homeless single people. Homeless people sleeping on the streets in London are currently being housed directly into their own permanent homes or into privately leased flats. This does not prove that some homeless single people do not need the extra support a hostel can offer, but it does suggest that attempts to apply a universal set of rules to tackling single homelessness only undermine the complexity of the problem.

Definitions of single homelessness seem to revolve around whether it can be accepted as a real need. The increase in people sleeping on London's streets provoked an outcry that this was unacceptable in a developed country like Britain. Such reactions disguise a confusion as to whether this is because people sleeping out cause obstruction to others or because there is a genuine concern over housing needs. It has never been established whether there is enough public will to solve single homelessness rather than simply cope with it. Until there is sufficient general understanding of the many reasons why single people become homeless, there will be no pressure to provide the resources necessary to create enough temporary and permanent housing for single people who are currently homeless and those who are at risk of becoming so in the future.

## SIZING UP THE PROBLEM OF SINGLE HOMELESSNESS

It is ironic that people who are single and homeless can be the most visible and invisible of people when it comes to counting up numbers. The problem of people sleeping out on the streets for the lack of anywhere else to go is plain for all to see, yet there are no official statistics kept on single homelessness. The lack of such records has been a major factor in preventing the development of a long-term strategy for dealing with single homelessness. Any figures compiled quickly become out-of-date. The lack of a major, objective assessment of the scale of single homelessness only adds to the sense that it is a problem too vague and wide-ranging to be capable of solution.

Surveys that have taken place are usually locally based. In London the only recent surveys were carried out in 1989. The first survey, by the London Research Centre on behalf of the Single Homeless in London Working Party (SHIL) (London Research Centre 1991), relied upon questionnaires sent to voluntary hostel and housing projects in London. The second survey, by the University of Surrey for the Salvation Army (Canter *et al.* 1989), involved a count of homeless people on the streets as well as an estimate of hostel places. The figures produced were:

| | | |
|---|---|---|
| SHIL | 13,500 | – Hostels |
| | 10–12,000 | – Short-life |
| | 19,000 | – Squatting |
| | 4–5,000 | – Bed & Breakfast |
| | 3,000 | – Sleeping Out |
| | 49,500–52,500 | |
| Salvation Army | 75,000 | – Total |

So, two surveys carried out in the same year still produced figures differing by 22,500 or 30 per cent. Figures are particularly difficult to establish for people sleeping out because of their mobility, and the problem that they may simply not be on their 'patch' when the count is made. A headcount of homeless people sleeping out has been done as part of the 1991 Census, but this exercise has taken over a year's careful preparation and provided a figure of 1,500 people sleeping out, which may be an underestimate. In 1990 the problem of collecting any useful figures on single homelessness was acknowledged in the overview report *Homelessness in Britain* (Greve and Currie 1990) for the National Federation of Housing Associations (NFHA) by Professor John Greve. The only figures available on single homelessness were those compiled by SHIL.

Another way of assessing the problem is to look at the number of hostel bedspaces. In London there are 18,500 hostel bedspaces owned by housing associations alone, so the total figure including other voluntary and privately run hostels may just exceed 20,000. The SHIL survey published in the *Move-on Housing* report (London Research Centre 1989) took a 'snapshot' picture of hostel occupancy for one night in June 1989. This showed that hostels were about 80 per cent full. The estimates of single homeless people described above are based on people who are visibly homeless, either sleeping on the streets or living in a temporary hostel. It is much more difficult to assess the number of people living as a 'concealed' household by sharing accommodation with a friend or family. The only indicators of the likely level of need are estimates made in the London Housing Survey 1986. This suggested that 180,000 people were living as concealed households and were therefore 'hidden homeless'.

## SINGLE HOMELESSNESS AND HOUSING POLICY

In assessing the effect of national housing policy on single homelessness, it is clear that no such policy has been specifically aimed at the problem. In spite of all the attention focused on housing in the past three to four years with the 1988 Housing Act, the needs of homeless single people have not been addressed. Single homeless people have experienced the consequences of national housing policy rather than been its beneficiaries. The only semblance of a national policy aimed at single homelessness has been the review of DSS Resettlement Units which began with the closure and replacement of the Camberwell Resettlement Unit in 1985. However, even this national programme is floundering through lack of funding and of any clear plan for how any new housing developed will meet the needs of homeless single people across the country.

Despite the continued growth in the number of single-person households, housing for single people is still regarded as marginal. In London, single people made up 22 per cent of all households in 1971.[1] This had increased to 26 per cent by 1981 and the London Research Centre predicts that this proportion will increase to 31 per cent by 2001. However, the focus of national housing policy has remained firmly on families.

Nevertheless, national housing policy has had a significant effect on single homelessness in five main ways:

- promotion of owner-occupation
- changes in private rented sector
- changes in housing role of local authorities
- changing demands upon housing associations
- changes in role of housing for people also in need of care and support.

## PROMOTION OF OWNER-OCCUPATION

The vigorous promotion of owner-occupation has had two major effects on single homelessness. The first, most obvious result has been to price much of the housing available out of the reach of many single people, reducing their housing options. The high level of house prices is well known, but it is worth comparing this with income levels to show how far out of reach home ownership is for homeless single people. In the second quarter of 1990,[2] the average price for a one-bedroom flat in London was £63,700; the lowest price for a one-bedroom flat was £47,000. Someone taking out a 95 per cent mortgage on £47,000 would need to pay a deposit of £2,350, or a deposit of £4,700 on a 90 per cent mortgage. The New Earnings Survey 1989 showed that 49 per cent of full-time workers in London earned less than £230 per week. Allowing for 10 per cent wage rise into 1990, these people would still earn less than the £14,300 per annum required for the £47,000 mortgage.

Second, emphasis on owner-occupation has further marginalized those people who have to rely on rented housing. Increasingly, this is regarded as a 'second-class option'. Consequently, as rented housing is often the only choice for many single people, the promotion of home ownership has further distanced the problem of single homelessness from the mainstream of housing policy.

## CHANGES IN THE PRIVATE RENTED SECTOR

More and more, the private rented sector is the only real option for single people. The decline of this sector is well documented, as are the possible reasons for this, although opinions concerning the causes vary. It is not proposed to go into detail about these here, but instead to examine what housing choice private renting offers to someone who is single and homeless.

It provides limited choice, in fact, because the amount of private rented housing has decreased and it has also become less affordable for people on low incomes. In London the private rented sector has been declining at a rate of 7 per cent a year (London Research Centre 1988). Despite some evidence that private renting is increasing in some areas, overall the trend is downwards. Any present increase seems linked to leasing arrangements set up by local authorities to help with the housing of statutorily homeless people, usually families.

The affordability of renting is more difficult to pin down accurately. Research carried out by the London Housing Unit on rents advertised in the London *Evening Standard* suggest weekly rents for one-bed accommodation of between £65 and £120 per week in mid-1990. Obviously advertisements in the paper cover a wide range of accommodation, but it does indicate that private renting is not a cheap option.

Along with home ownership, encouragement of private renting has been actively pursued by government, particularly for people who cannot afford home ownership. Only recently, the government announced a new pilot project to encourage more private landlords to work in partnership with housing associations and bring their empty (private) properties back into housing use.

The promotion of private renting as a housing choice for people on low incomes has depended on the support of housing benefit. Rents could rise because housing benefit would be available to bridge the gap for people on low incomes. This works well as long as:

- housing benefit is able to cover the rent cost
- someone receiving housing benefit is not working and so is receiving full income support.

If housing benefit cannot meet the full cost of the rent, the difference has to be met by the tenant. This can arise because rent officers can determine a rent on a property which is judged to be reasonable. Local authorities have to pay housing benefit only on the 'determined' rent level: any rent above this, and payment of additional housing benefit by the local authority to meet the gap is discretionary.

To receive full housing benefit it is also necessary to be on full state benefit. Any income earned above is deducted at a rate of 65 pence in the pound. Anyone earning but on a low wage will have to meet a significant part of their rent costs before receiving any housing benefit.

## CHANGES IN THE HOUSING ROLE OF LOCAL AUTHORITIES

As local authorities have no statutory duty to house the majority of homeless single people, the effect of changes in their role regarding single homelessness is again characterized by distance. The amount of help given to homeless single people has been discretionary and so varies considerably. The type of help provided is usually in the form of advice to individual applicants for housing; operating their own services such as hostels; or, more usually, funding other organizations to provide services. Services for homeless people are normally only a small element of a local authority's housing operation and are vulnerable to cuts if the authority's main housing service requires more resources.

The effects of recent changes in local authority housing on single homelessness are therefore more difficult to perceive than effects on family housing. This causes problems for organizations seeking to raise the effects of policy and legislative changes on homeless single people.

Changes in the local authority housing role have had implications for single homelessness because there has been an increasing pressure both on local authority housing stock and on local housing finance. The pressure on housing stock has been well documented. Council house building has decreased significantly. The number of homes built by local authorities in London fell every year in the 1980s. Provisional information for 1990 shows fewer than 400 new housing starts by London boroughs that year (London Research Centre 1991). Over the three years 1987 to 1990 the number of new local authority homes in London never exceeded 2,000, compared to an annual total of approximately 15,000 homes in 1980. Nationally, local authority house completions dropped by 82 per cent between 1980 and 1990, from 78,000 to 13,980.

Promotion of right-to-buy has depleted the housing stock available for rent without the loss being compensated by new building, by either local authorities or housing associations. Increases in statutory homelessness have put local authorities under great pressure to use the majority of their housing resources for housing families. Small-sized council accommodation, such as one-bedroom flats or bedsits, which was previously available to single homeless people, is now being used for homeless families in preference to bed and breakfast accommodation. This can be seen in the reduction of 'move-on' housing offered by local authorities to housing agencies for housing single homeless people from hostels. Financially, the 1989 Local Government and Housing Act has resulted in tighter controls on local authorities' housing spending via the Housing Revenue Account. This cannot be subsidized by the community charge and must be kept in balance. Local authority rents have risen in order to achieve this. Council housing has therefore not only become a reduced option for single homeless people but it has also become more expensive.

Pressures on resources for mainstream housing services have resulted in less funding being available for single homelessness. This can be seen in the reduction or freezing of grants to voluntary housing agencies and housing associations managing and developing housing for single people. In some instances, local authorities have disbanded or withdrawn their support from forums in their areas looking at special needs housing because of a lack of resources.

These are tangible effects of changes in local authority housing, but they remain marginal because there is no duty on authorities to monitor them and currently no means available for doing so. There is one area in which the way local authorities have already been approaching single homelessness can, in fact, contribute to a major current change in local authority housing policy generally. One of the aims of the 1988 Housing Act and 1989 Local Government and Housing Act was to encourage local authorities to take on an enabling rather than a providing role in relation to housing. As services for single homeless people have largely been developed by local authorities funding other organizations, usually voluntary housing agencies or housing associations, the enabling role is already well established. To develop it further, local authorities are examining their partnerships with agencies and housing associations which have traditionally helped develop housing for single homeless people.

## CHANGING DEMANDS UPON HOUSING ASSOCIATIONS

Housing associations have been traditional, if small, providers of housing for single homeless people. Housing associations developed to meet housing need which could not be filled by a local authority. Associations thus have a role as innovators in identifying and helping the majority of single homeless people who fall outside the categories of statutorily homeless for whom the local authority has responsibility. Homes developed for single homeless people vary widely, from hostels and shared houses to self-contained flats and bedsits.

Housing associations are therefore important providers of housing for homeless single people, although their housing stock is small in comparison with that of local authorities. In 1990, after a decade of substantial central government and local government investment in special needs housing, London housing associations owned 18,000 hostel bedspaces, half the national total, yet the number of people single and homeless in London was still estimated at between 50,000 and 75,000.

Changes in the role of housing associations have been significant for single homelessness. The 1988 Housing Act has resulted in housing associations becoming the main developers of rented housing for people on low incomes, in place of local authorities. Consequently, associations now have a vital role in assisting local authorities to house homeless families. The Housing Corporation, responsible for funding and monitoring housing associations, has been set by government to target 50 per cent of its funding at tackling homelessness. Sixty per cent of this, however, is to be aimed at statutorily homelessness, mainly that of homeless families.

The effect of this concentration of housing association resources on statutorily homeless people has been to freeze or reduce funding available for single homelessness. Another traditional source of housing for single people is therefore under pressure.

Changes in the financing of housing associations have also raised concerns over their ability to continue developing housing for single homeless people on a scale needed to meet demand. The 1988 Housing Act introduced the use of private finance to supplement grants to housing associations for developing homes for people in housing need. Housing associations now have to find other forms of funding, e.g. corporate finance, rather than rely on 100 per cent funding from the Housing Corporation (a government body which distributes funding to housing association projects).

Using private finance has exposed housing associations to greater risk, and so they have had to assess carefully which housing schemes to develop. Housing for single homeless people, particularly hostel provision, is susceptible to greater financial risk, because of both the complexity of development and the revenue finance needed to support the housing management costs. Consequently, associations have had to assess special needs housing schemes carefully to ensure that private finance can be raised and that developing a scheme will not place the association at risk.

More positively, the changes introduced by the 1988 Housing Act highlighted the need for financing of special needs housing to be brought into line with the funding of mainstream housing for housing associations. Capital funding for developing special needs housing has now been put on the same basis as mainstream housing. More importantly, the introduction of the new system of revenue funding to support the extra housing management costs of special needs housing enables associations to develop self-contained as well as shared accommodation. The new Special Needs Management Allowance (SNMA) will hopefully enable associations to develop a wider range of special needs housing to meet specific needs.

## SINGLE HOMELESSNESS AND COMMUNITY CARE

Changes in other areas of government policy in the care and support services beyond housing have had significant effects for homeless single people. These are considered in more detail later, so will not be examined closely here. However, it is essential to understand how the role of housing is perceived for single people who are both homeless and in need of some form of care.

One view of the role of housing in providing care for people within the community was set out in the Griffiths Report: *Community Care: An Agenda for Action* (Griffiths 1988). Housing was accorded only a minor role, treated in its most basic form as simply providing the 'bricks and mortar'. Housing was secondary to the care and support services and not acknowledged as having a contribution to make towards the needs of someone requiring support.

Not surprisingly, housing professionals, particularly from voluntary agencies and housing associations, disagreed with this view. In 1989 the National Federation of Housing Associations (NFHA) published *Housing: The Foundation of Community Care* which proposed that housing was the basis for providing a complete service to people with care needs.

Both views demonstrate the confusion that surrounds the role of housing for people with care needs. The fact that many single homeless people are in need of some form of care or support has been well established. It has been acknowledged by central government in their establishment of a programme targeted at helping homeless mentally ill people in central London. The Department of Health is developing this programme on estimates of 1,000 single people sleeping rough in London who are mentally ill.

Confusion over the role of housing for single homeless people in need of care has led to a range of housing being developed. Supported housing can vary from projects providing intensive support with a structured care programme to those with care services provided externally according to the needs of the individual. For someone who is single and homeless, it can often be pot luck as to what type of service he or she receives, and can depend on which agency they approach and where they are based.

It can also be difficult for supported housing services to account for changes in care needed by someone. Care requirements, particularly for people who have a mental illness, can fluctuate considerably, and it can be difficult to provide individuals with a flexible level of care, especially where housing is central to ensuring the care is provided.

The overall effect of community care changes has also been to affect single homeless people from a distance. Care and support issues have been considered in detail, but not the equally important needs arising from being homeless. Housing and care services have therefore been grafted together in the absence of a clear policy direction, resulting in many different forms of supported housing.

## SINGLE HOMELESSNESS AND BENEFITS

Single homeless people have experienced significant change as a result of the many developments in the social security benefit system over the past ten years. Details of these are not going to be listed here as they would take up too much space: only the broad implications of changes will be set out.

It is easy to lose sight of the major effects of benefit changes for homeless single people within the mass of detailed developments that have taken place. For many, benefits are still the only source of money with which to pay the rent and bills and buy food and clothes. Without this income, hostel projects could not function as they would receive no rent. The individual and the services providing for his or her needs are both crucially dependent upon the benefits system. Any change, no matter how small, in the way such benefits apply affects both homeless people and hostels.

Again, the common theme of provision for single homeless people being brought into line with mainstream services without sufficient thought of the implications is evident. The key benefit change which has been introduced was the transfer of all hostel residents from support payments for 'Board and Lodging' to a combination of housing benefit and income support. The board and lodging payment structure was geared to the life in shared housing, even though there was a ceiling on the payment level for four years until the system changed in 1989. It has been complicated to adapt the combination of housing benefit and income support to meet the needs of a single homeless person living in a temporary hostel. For example, housing benefit accounts for the cost of heating and lighting a communal area in the hostel, but the cost of these in a resident's room can be met only from a person's income support payment. Such negotiations have been difficult for projects to deal with, involving discussions with the Department of Social Security, the local authority and the resident. Time taken in such discussion can result in less opportunity for developing better services within the hostel. Hostel projects have had to invest more in training staff to enable them to deal with these changes and also spend time chasing the prompt payment of both housing benefit and income support.

Justification of this very significant change in benefit is difficult to untangle. The Department of Social Security commissioned research which demonstrated that support services within hostels funded partly by board and lodging payments were not essential, and so need not be resourced by the department. As a result of a rigorous campaign by voluntary agencies and housing associations some flexibility was obtained, and a complex system of transitional protection funding was introduced for both individual homeless people and voluntary agencies. This resulted in the ludicrous situation of homeless people entering a hostel after 9 October 1989 being paid less in benefits than someone who had started living in the hostel on 8 October.

Benefit changes affecting young people have been much publicized. Since September 1988, 16- and 17-year-olds are not entitled to income support and 18–25-year-olds receive a lower level of both housing benefit and income support. Such constraints cause considerable problems in finding either stable temporary or permanent housing. It is difficult to see what distinguishes the costs of housing for a 22-year-old from those of someone who is 25. Research by voluntary agencies has shown that many of the young single homeless people approaching them have left care or are unable to return home for fear of abuse or because their relationship with parents has completely broken down.

The introduction of the Social Fund has also caused problems for single homeless people trying to establish a permanent home. Prior to the Social Fund, it was possible to receive a grant towards the costs of setting up a permanent home, essential for buying expensive but necessary items such as a cooker or bed. Some funding is still available in this form via community care grants, but these are limited and the practice of granting them can vary. Again, success is dependent upon the skills of the voluntary agency negotiating on behalf of someone who is homeless. The Social Fund enables people to apply for loans, but repayments can be difficult for people on low wages and granting of a loan can depend on whether the local social security office has sufficient money available.

Changes in benefits have affected single homeless people by becoming more complicated, restrictive and elusive. There has been no constructive approach to considering how benefits could be best used to support long-term housing solutions for homeless single people.

## SINGLE HOMELESSNESS AND HEALTH POLICY

Changes in the National Health Service and their effects on homeless single people are the central issues addressed in this book. These have been considered last in the chapter in order to set them against the many other developments which have affected homeless single people in recent years. Points raised here will be brief as the detail is provided in later chapters.

Reviews of both the National Health Service and community care services have been significant for homeless single people. Again, it is difficult to measure this in absolute terms because, in the same way that there are no measures of single homelessness, there is no easy means of recording how homeless single people use the health services. The marginalization of homeless single people is reinforced once more.

Debate about the best means of ensuring that health services are available to homeless single people has centred around the issue of whether it is best to secure access to mainstream health services or to provide specific, separate services. The view supporting access to mainstream services is a difficult one to counter. The PSI Report *Health Care for Single Homeless People* (Allen and Williams 1989) observed that 'There is an enormous danger that special services provided by special teams only serve to further marginalise people who are already operating on the borders of society.' The report made no firm recommendations that health provision for homeless single people should be developed via mainstream services, but two other reports published at the time strongly recommended this case. These were *Primary Health Care for Homeless Single People in London: A Strategic Approach* (SHIL 1987) and *From the Margins to the Mainstream* (Stern *et al.* 1989).

However, the lack of adequate mainstream health care services available to homeless single people has encouraged the development of more specific, separate services. Housing projects arrange for a doctor's surgery to be held in the project or for a nurse's services to be available. The debate is therefore a very current live issue.

One of the main concerns underlying the drive to secure greater access to mainstream health services is to avoid stereotyping the health needs of homeless single people. Studies of health requirements have often focused on problems such as alcohol or drug abuse, chronic diseases such as bronchitis or tuberculosis and mental illness. It has been more difficult to achieve an understanding of the overall health needs of people who are homeless and single. The PSI report usefully acknowledged that 'the way in which the health problems of the homeless were seen to differ from those of the general population was largely one of degree rather than substance'. The problems of gaining a wider acceptance for this in light of the health service reforms are considered below.

General practitioner services are still key in securing access to other parts of the Health Service, including mental health provision, as well as providing primary health care. It is well established that some GPs are reluctant to take on single homeless people as patients and, as a result, single homeless people are often reluctant to register. The pilot projects in Camden and East London in the mid-1980s discovered that, although single homeless people would use the primary health care services provided by their teams, they would be reluctant to go and register with other local GPs, preferring to use a service they were familiar with. Issues arising from this basic requirement for access to health services have not been fully researched. The PSI report quoted above was commissioned to evaluate the pilot projects and considered registration with GPs. However, the figures produced on this matter had little meaning and the report did not look in any depth at reasons for not registering with GPs.

Even if this primary service was more widely available to homeless single people, changes in Health Service legislation may discourage GPs from accepting them as patients. The introduction of practice budgets and limitations on funding for prescription treatments may increase GPs' reluctance to take on single homeless people if they are perceived as potentially awkward and expensive patients. Housing agencies also expressed concern that increase in capitation fees for GPs would discourage GPs from treating single homeless people who may have awkward or long-term conditions requiring a lot of time and attention. The new capitation fees would encourage GPs to see more patients, but within a shorter time scale.

Continuity of care is probably as important for many homeless single people as gaining access to health services. The lack of any firm basis of primary health care results in a patchy service in other areas of health. The problem of homeless single people being discharged from hospital with nowhere to go is widely known. Someone who is homeless and single may receive substantial treatment in one district health authority, then be rehoused in another district and find it difficult to secure funding from the district for health care. The issues of lack of any clear responsibility for providing or planning health services for homeless single people are apparent in a similar way to the lack of any direct housing responsibility. Again, homeless single people are simply one of many competing priorities for funds, which fact, combined with a lack of any locatable responsibility, indicates that their needs will continue to be poorly considered.

As in the recent development of housing legislation, homeless single people have not been identified as requiring particular consideration yet the result of Health Service and community care reforms could be significant. The problem is intensified by the inability to measure the effects of these changes: resources are hard-pressed and it is unlikely that district health authorities will be able or willing to commission specific research in this area.

## SINGLE HOMELESSNESS IN LONDON: HOW POLICY HAS DEVELOPED

Changes affecting homeless single people have not only been brought about by legislation and government policy. Development has also taken place in the way that voluntary agencies, housing associations and statutory organizations have approached the problem of single homelessness. These changes have been particularly noticeable in London where the majority of housing for homeless single people has been developed.

Changes in London have been influenced partly by the type of funding that has been available, but also by the experience of implementing major hostel closure and replacement programmes. In London there has also been a unique combination of funding, service delivery and policy development in a joint working party of statutory and voluntary organizations. The Single Homeless in London Working Party (SHIL) has now been running for fourteen years and still maintains its joint statutory/voluntary membership and all-party political support from London boroughs.

Development of temporary and permanent housing for single homeless people in London has been largely affected by the need to deal with a number of closures of large, institutional-style hostels and night-shelters in the early 1980s. These closures, particularly that of the DHSS-owned Camberwell Resettlement Unit, influenced national policy on development of housing for single homeless people. The hostels were very large (Camberwell provided 1,000 bedspaces in the early 1980s) and were often for men only. Even today, such emergency housing is in short supply for single homeless women, with only 433 bedspaces compared to 1,480 available for men (SHIL 1991). Many of the men in the Camberwell hostel had been resident for many years, and this was the case in several other similar large hostels.

The drive to close and replace the Camberwell hostel, and the Rowton hostels soon after, also followed the announcement of the government's 'Hostels Initiative' in 1981. This encouraged housing associations to develop hostels for single homeless people. A pattern of partnership arrangements was established between housing associations and voluntary agencies for the associations to build the hostels and the agencies to manage them. Government encouraged this by providing capital funding to associations via the Housing Corporation, and some revenue funding through a grant known as Hostel Deficit Grant. Top-up revenue grants were provided by a mixture of organizations, principally the GLC and London boroughs and other government departments such as the DHSS and Home Office. In London, this funding and development of hostels were brought together and further promoted by SHIL.

The structures to develop new hostels were therefore in place when the issue of replacing London's other large hostels arose. Replacement of the hostels was heavily influenced by the need to deal with the many men living in them so it was inevitable that the 'replacement' projects were largely developed around the needs of the hostel residents. The high degree of institutionalization amongst the men led to a range of hostel services being developed, providing 'high', 'medium' or 'low' care according to need.

Hostel projects were generally regarded as temporary housing from where a resident would move on to permanent housing once his or her initial needs had been dealt with. This was possible in a smaller hostel or shared housing project as there was less danger of someone becoming institutionalized. The higher levels of staffing also enabled more support to be given on an individual basis to hostel residents.

At that time, the model of the very large hostel was universally rejected by statutory and voluntary agencies as being unsuitable for single homeless people. New proposals for emergency hostels to replace Camberwell proposed a maximum number of between thirty and thirty-six bedspaces.

With the combination of the Hostels Initiative and major programmes to close and replace large hostels in London, new hostel and shared housing development rapidly increased. There are now over 18,000 hostel bedspaces owned by housing associations in London, representing 40 per cent of the national total.

The rapid development of hostel provision in London, continually supported by the funding available to operate it, had two main results. It encouraged development of a great diversity of hostels targeted at a range of needs and groups of homeless single people. It also reinforced the perception of the hostel as a necessary stage in resolving a single person's homelessness: direct rehousing into permanent accommodation was not given a high profile.

The development of more hostel projects encouraged the increasing co-ordination of hostel and shared housing activity amongst voluntary agencies. Support agencies such as the Special Needs Housing

Advisory Service (SNHAS) now SITRA and other co-ordinating forums helped to focus debate amongst agencies on how best to develop future services for single homeless people.

The campaign to develop more permanent housing was largely the work of the voluntary agencies, taken up by SHIL and culminating in the *Move-On Housing* report of 1989. The debate around move-on housing concentrated on the need to free up places in temporary hostels and enable residents to 'move-on' to permanent homes. The term 'move-on' has been much discussed, as, although it describes the need for hostel residents to have access to forms of permanent housing, it excludes the possibility of single homeless people being housed directly into a permanent home.

Recent initiatives on single homlessness in London have made it clear that permanent housing is an issue. The initial 'Rooflessness Initiative' announced in 1990/91 by the then Housing Minister Michael Spicer enabled permanent housing to be developed alongside schemes offering emergency, night-shelter type housing. This was important as it provided single people on the streets the possibility of direct access to permanent housing. The more substantial programme of single homeless initiatives running from 1991 to 1993 has seen £50 million invested in permanent housing for single people. Again, the voice of voluntary agencies has been influential is shaping the choice of housing schemes. At first it was thought that most of the money should be used to produce permanent self-contained homes. After discussion with voluntary agencies working with single people sleeping on the street of central London, some of the money was given to schemes which could also provide support within permanent housing. The aim was shifted to enable a greater choice of permanent housing to be made available.

The description of changes in responses to single homelessness outlined above is necessarily broad and does not do justice to the immense variety of voluntary projects which have been set up to help meet a single increasing need. What it does show, hopefully, is that housing providers are now looking at developing more choice for someone who is single and homeless, in both temporary and permanent housing terms.

## CONCLUSION

The effects of recent social policy in housing, health, community care and welfare benefits have been generally to marginalize homeless single people. There has been no specific social policy aimed directly at single homelessness, except perhaps for benefit changes for 16–25-year-olds. However, it is clear that the major changes which have been taking place in all these social policy areas have had a very significant effect upon single homeless people. Often, these have taken place with only limited consultation with voluntary organizations representing the case of single homeless people, particularly in areas outside housing such as health.

Single homeless people are just as affected by major legislative change in social policy areas as people who are housed. The recent government initiatives focused on single homelessness in Central London are demonstrating that the mainstream housing and other support services must be strengthened to provide for their needs. A recent study of hostel providers and residents by the University of Salford concluded that:

> the major problems of the homeless were simply and primarily lack of accommodation, low income and unemployment rather than any identifiable 'special Need'.
>
> (Garside *et al.* 1991: 32)

These are problems which can affect everyone. It is useful to bear this in mind when considering single homeless people, as too often they are seen as a group apart instead of as people who simply face enormous problems in finding a permanent home.

## NOTES

1 London Research Centre, from OPCS Censuses 1971 and 1981, p. 9.
2 Halifax Building Society, House Price Data, p. 10.

## REFERENCES

Allen, I. and Williams, S. (1989) *Health Care for Single Homeless People*, London: Policy Studies Institute, p. 28.

Canter, D. *et al.* (1989) *The Faces of Homelessness in London: Interim Report to the Salvation Army*, Department of Psychology University of Surrey, p. 6.

Garside, P.L., Grimshaw, R.W. and Ward, F.W. (1991) *Managing Accommodation: the Experience of Providers and Residents*, Department of Environmental Health and Housing University of Salford (reviewed in *Housing Review* Sept/Oct), p. 32.

Greve, J. and Currie, E. (1990) *Homelessness in Britain*, Joseph Rowntree Memorial Trust, p. 7.

Griffiths, R. (1988) *Community Care: an Agenda for Action*, a report to the Secretary of State for Social Services, p. 18.

LRC (1988) *Access to Housing in London*, a report based on the results of the London Housing Survey 1986/7, London Research Centre, p. 11.

LRC (1989) *Move-On Housing*, NFHA Research Report 4 SHIL, p. 6.

LRC (1991) *London Housing Statistics 1990/91*, London Research Centre, p. 13.

NFHA (1989) *Housing: the Foundation of Community Care*, National Federation of Housing Associations, p. 19.

SHIL (1987) *Primary Health Care for Homeless Single People in London: a Strategic Approach*, SHIL, p. 29.

SHIL (1991) 'Direct access statistics', p. 24.

Stern, R. *et al.* (1989) *From the Margins to the Mainstream*, SHHARP, p. 29.

# 2 Access to health care

*Kevin Fisher and John Collins*

> . . . homeless people in particular may find it difficult to use the NHS.
>
> (Royal Commission on the NHS 1979)

The difficulties that many single homeless men and women have faced in obtaining access to health care have often been viewed by the public and service providers alike as 'their problem' or 'their fault'. Stereotypical images, said to reflect the attributes and characteristics of the homeless person, are invoked to justify this assertion. Put simply, it is suggested that homeless people find it difficult to get access to health care because they are too smelly, too dirty and often too drunk. They frighten other patients and sometimes staff, they are too mobile and they do not keep appointments. Health problems become pathology and pathology is perceived as having deviant overtones, as the following extract from a report submitted to the Department of Health illustrates:

> Pathology among the single homeless is perhaps more apparent as deviant behaviour than as physical illness. Very heavy drinking is extremely common, as also is excessive gambling – in many cases, these activities are quite clearly beyond the individual's control. One of the doctors consulted felt that almost all of the homeless men he had seen had serious personality problems and some were overtly psychotic.
>
> (NFA 1974)

By focusing on the individual, such descriptions of the problem act as a useful means of distracting attention from structural explanations of both the problems of homelessness and the obtaining of health care. In his book *Blaming the Victim*, Ryan describes this process:

> All this happens so smoothly that it seems downright rational. First identify a social problem. Second, study those affected by the

problem and discover in what ways they are different from the rest of us as a consequence of deprivation and injustice. Third, define the difference as the cause of the social problem itself. Finally, of course assign a government bureaucrat to invent a humanitarian programme to correct the differences.

(Ryan 1971: 8–9)

It becomes all to easy to forget that the problem of access to health care is a by-product of a problem of access to affordable accommodation.

## THE ENVIRONMENTAL AND SOCIAL CONTEXT

A number of studies (Laidlaw 1955; Scott *et al.* 1966; McCrory 1975; Toon 1985; Stern *et al.* 1989) from the mid-1950s onwards have drawn attention to the increased vulnerability of single homeless men and women to certain forms of ill health. Laidlaw's survey of the state of health of the residents of Glasgow common lodging houses is a catalogue of previously undiagnosed and untreated conditions which revealed an astonishing level of acceptance of chronic ill health both among the residents of the lodging houses and by their wardens. For example, the seven cases of cancer he diagnosed were all subsequently admitted to hospital. Two were found to be in a terminal condition. 'Neither of these had previously sought medical advice, and it was not until they were unable to rise from their bunks that the superintendent became aware that they were ill' (Laidlaw 1955).

Twenty-five years later *Community Care* reported the death of Arthur Stevens of chronic bronchitis and emphysema in a South London hostel. Arthur had been ill for nine months but had suffered from homelessness for twelve years. When he was found dead he weighed just over 6 stone and was thought to be aged between 45 and 50. The pathologist noted that he looked 'rather wasted, far older than his stated age' (Harrington 1980). The staff in the hostel had noticed that he did not look well but did little or nothing to help him seek medical attention. He died without ever seeing a doctor.

These examples point to a pivotal cause of the high level of ill health among the single homeless – the environmental and social context in which they exist. Thus the most vulnerable and most deprived live their lives in conditions of squalor and poverty of Dickensian proportions. A spokesperson for CHAR described the hostel in which Arthur Stevens died as 'a risk to the health, safety and welfare of the people who have to live there. The premises have no heating, the amenities are below minimum legal standards and are in such a state of disrepair that they are unfit for human habitation' (Harrington 1980). This hostel remained open until 1990 and at the time of writing has been reopened in a slightly improved condition, as part of a government initiative to provide direct access accommodation to single homeless men.

Other studies have pointed to the high incidence of certain conditions among some sections of the homeless population. McCrory, writing in 1975, found that the occurrence of TB among Edinburgh's lodging house population was five times greater than the city average. In 1983 the *Observer* reported that TB was endemic in another London hostel, where the rate of TB infection among the resident population was one hundred times that of the national average. While the incidence of TB is now dropping among the homeless as some of the large hostels have been closed down, it was the unsanitary conditions, overcrowding, a poor diet and alcohol abuse which encouraged the prevalence of this disease. Hostel closures have meant that there is now a shortage of direct access provision in metropolitan areas. Some ex-residents and others within the homeless milieu have been forced to exchange the squalor of the hostel for the destitution of the street with its own attendant dangers.

Poverty and squalor are not the only factors which underlie many homeless people's experience. Just as debilitating is the stigma which handicaps, marginalizes and creates barriers. Here inequality is at its most extreme. Poor clothing and the difficulty of maintaining personal hygiene lead many homeless people to feel marginal or deviant. One man, asked if his health had deteriorated since he became homeless, replied:

> Yes it did. Not only my health but I suppose your nerves come into it. You become like a bag of nerves. You're not settled, you're afraid all the time. You don't sleep properly unless you're really exhausted, you know, through roaming about all day. Your feet ache. Your whole body aches and you just say I'll kip down here for the night. You don't sleep properly. You're a bag of nerves and uncomfortable. You get up the next morning, you look around you people passing you by. If you've any shame in you at all you're frightened to look them in the face because they know very well that you're one of those sleeping rough. They look down on you.
>
> (Fisher 1989)

It comes as no surprise that some single homeless people choose to avoid the experience of being peered at or shunned in doctors' waiting-rooms or clinics.

## ACCESS TO HEALTH CARE

**Primary care**

The Acheson Report said of GPs 'they lie at the heart of a good and effective primary health care service for the great majority of people and the source of referral to other professionals and agencies' (Acheson 1981). Indeed it is a matter of statute that every citizen has a right to register with a general medical practitioner, but one of the quirks of the independent contractor status of GPs within the NHS is that: unless assigned to his/her 'list' by a Family Health Services Authority (FHSA) (and then only for a period of three months), no GP has an obligation to accept responsibility for an individual requesting registration. This anomaly has been present since the inception of the NHS in 1948. It has been beneficial since it gave rise to the need for registration in order to assess payments to GPs and this mechanism allows for the medical record to pass from GP to GP throughout life, facilitating medical care – a situation unique in the world.

The assignment mechanisms mentioned, whereby a GP can be obliged to register (for three months) a named patient, are not a useful recourse for homeless people for several reasons. First, they are slow and unwieldy, relying on assignment sub-committees of the FHSA, (reference to these is generally made by social workers on behalf of families with children). Second, self-advocacy skills and assertiveness are required to make them work and homeless people commonly have insufficient self-esteem to achieve this. Finally, there is a common understanding that an 'unwilling' GP may be an unhelpful one.

Not all GPs are unwilling to register and care for homeless people. Practical administrative obstacles to achieving this mean that many who do are underpaid for their work. It is important to note that the social milieu of modern medical practice – often in busy health centres with appointment systems, computers and busy waiting areas – is seen as off-putting by some homeless people, so that they seek out other avenues to care or struggle on without it. The development of outreach initiatives (Brickner *et al.* 1986) and health advocacy work among homeless people (personal communications 1991 PCHP)[1] are important models in this regard. Added to this are bureaucratic difficulties. Some FHSAs won't accept patient registration for addressless people.

*Types of registration*

There are three main ways by which an NHS GP may receive payment for patient care:

### Permanent registration (usually abbreviated to Registration)

Patients resident in the GP's FHS area for three months or more, or intending to be so, are registered as permanent patients. Commonly GPs will accept patients only within a smaller 'practice' area (which in inner cities extends often no more than a half-mile radius from their surgeries). Permanent registration means that a GP contracts to provide twenty-four-hour cover for that patient, an NHS medical card is issued to the patient and the GP will, in due course, usually receive previous medical records from the patient's last known GP (England/Scotland and Wales only).

### Temporary registration

This allows a person to be treated for a period of up to three months and should apply only if a person is intending to remain in the FHS area for less than this time. (Temporary registration can, however, be extended for up to six months in any one year or transferred to permanent registration after three months.) There are three important differences between temporary and permanent registration:

a) Temporary registration does not lead to the transfer of medical records from previous GP(s). This disadvantages the doctor (and the patient) and impairs continuity of care.
b) A medical card is not issued to temporary patients – in fact the patient has no record of this arrangement.
c) Homeless people often perceive temporary registration as an inferior arrangement which enhances suspicion of the doctor's motives and reinforces poor self-esteem.

It is well worth noting that this mechanism was created not to serve the needs of homeless people but mainly to provide care for holiday makers, visitors and those working away from home and presumes permanent registration is effective with a doctor elsewhere in the country.

### Emergency treatment

This is worth mentioning only because homeless people of no fixed abode are commonly treated under this arrangement. Again, the patient has no record but the mechanism is designed for sudden emergencies/accidents afflicting persons who are visiting or resident within the FHS area for less than twenty-four hours only. The doctor's responsibility is limited to that period. It is generally inappropriate for homeless people to be treated under this arrangement just because their exact whereabouts within a locality are undefined.

None of these points would be worth exploring if the NHS GP service was salaried and/or patch-based with defined geographical responsibilities. There are many aspects to the debate about the relative merits of this, as opposed to existing arrangements, which are inappropriate to pursue here. Suffice it to say that, from the point of view of homeless, mobile or addressless people, statutory primary medical care would probably be easier to obtain under such a system.

A number of commentators have described general practitioners as the 'gatekeepers' of the health service, determining need and regulating demand. Foster, in her book *Access to Welfare*, describes how GPs use two distinct gatekeeping strategies. 'Firstly they control patients' access to their own time, attention and expertise. Second they largely control patients' access to a range of health care resources, including prescribed drugs and medicines and most hospital and consultant services' (Foster 1983).

While gatekeeping can be viewed as both a legitimate and a necessary function it does mean that GPs are entitled, without reason, to refuse registration and may use this entitlement to avoid taking on the care of people whom they, or their existing patients, perceive to be difficult, demanding, disruptive or dishevelled.

For example, Taylor reported in 1987 that, in inner-city Liverpool, several residential hostels for people with mental health problems were having difficulty in gaining registration for their patients.

Reluctant GPs have been cited as the main reason why single homeless people have difficulties in getting access to health care. This was graphically illustrated by an enterprising experiment conducted by City and Hackney Community Health Council. They instructed 'Dick', described in an article by Mind as a 'bogus vagrant' (*Mind News* 1980), to attempt to register with six local GPs. In four out of six attempts Dick was refused permanent registration, temporary registration or emergency treatment.

A study by CHAR and ACHCEW (Association of Community Health Councils in England and Wales), based on a questionnaire sent to fourteen urban areas, found that 'difficulties were reported from all the areas surveyed in finding GPs willing to take on homeless people, even as temporary residents. Many thousands of homeless people have effectively no access to a local doctor' (ACHCEW/CHAR 1980).

In Manchester all twenty-eight practices within one mile of the city's main hostels and lodging houses were contacted. Although half were not prepared to collaborate, eighteen doctors from fourteen practices agreed to be interviewed about single homeless people as patients. All the GPs interviewed seemed to expect a homeless person to correspond to the 'down and out' stereotype: 'middle aged, usually unkempt and/or dirty; permanently wedded to an unstable lifestyle' (Manchester CHC 1980). In spite of the proximity of these GPs to a single homeless population of 15,000 only six of the practices contacted had any homeless patients on their list. Three of the practices said they refused to treat homeless people as a matter of policy. One doctor quoted in the report said that hostel residents, whom he described as 'those with half a dozen overcoats and a million lice', were 'never in one place for more than five minutes. They can use casualty departments' (Manchester CHC 1980).

On a more optimistic note the report stated that five GPs who had no single homeless patients said they would be willing to treat homeless people if they presented themselves:

> none of these five attempted to explain away the problems in terms of the inadequacy or wilful abuse of the homeless person. Indeed, three saw such problems as the consequence of a consistently poor environment, resulting in long term neglect that inevitably leads to both health breakdown and poor health expectations.
>
> (Manchester CHC 1980)

More recently, as part of a study of health care and single homelessness, researchers from the Policy Studies Institute interviewed thirty-four GPs who had surgeries in close proximity to two experimental health care projects for the homeless. Nearly all the GPs interviewed (82 per cent) felt that there were fundamental problems in permanently registering homeless people. One of the main obstacles they cited was the mobility of many of the homeless. Some GPs felt the problem was a bureaucratic one, that the Family Practitioner Committee would not allow them to register permanently someone who did not have an address (some will accept the use of other contact points, e.g. day centres). Others, however, linked mobility with financial considerations. As one GP pointed out:

> The problem is a logistical one. If we sign someone on to claim the

capitation fee and they've disappeared by the end of that quarter and registered with another GP, no matter how many times we have seen them we don't receive a penny. The hassle would be financial as well as administrative.

(Williams and Allen 1989)

These factors mean that, especially since the revised contractual arrangements for GPs introduced in April 1990, most GPs favour temporary registration or emergency treatment mechanisms when caring for homeless people. A majority of the GPs interviewed (75 per cent) made a distinction between people living in hostels and those who were sleeping out and a quarter of those interviewed said they would be prepared to register hostel residents permanently but not people living on the streets.

The problems of treating single homeless people were not confined to registration. A number of GPs mentioned the time factor. They felt that the everyday pressures of providing an adequate service did not allow them to give sufficient attention to the often more time consuming needs of their homeless patients.

Other GPs were worried about the reactions of their other patients whom they felt would be disturbed by the 'anti-social aspects of them, both behavioural and olfactory' (Williams and Allen 1989). Many GPs in urban areas fear an 'avalanche of need' emerging should they begin to accept homeless patients. The basic problems of homelessness are not soluble in or by the NHS: needs in the general practice population are already high (AGUDA 1990); secondary care services are over-burdened (BMA 1991); social work support for single people, especially alcohol abusers, is generally a low priority for local authority social services departments. All these factors contribute to an understandable 'avoidance' of the problems of homeless people by some doctors.

While the reluctance of general practitioners to register single homeless people is frequently cited as being the main barrier to access, recent empirical evidence would seem to indicate that this is only part of the equation. For their study, *From the Margins to the Main-stream: Collaboration in Planning Services with Single Homeless People*, the West Lambeth Priority Services Unit interviewed 312 homeless men and women whom they subsequently divided into accommodation groups. While the average level of registration for the whole survey population was 64 per cent there was a wide disparity between accommodation groups. Thus, while 83 per cent of project (supportive hostels) residents were registered, only 35 per cent of those sleeping out had their own GP.

The authors also looked at the level of registration in the Lambeth area in order to discover the extent to which people in the sample would have to travel in order to consult their GP. None of the people sleeping out were registered in the area while 71 per cent of people living in special projects were registered locally. When the study asked people who were not registered whether they had tried to register since becoming homeless, over 82 per cent said they had made no attempt. Only 7 per cent of the main sample said they had tried and failed. The twelve people who had tried to register but had failed were asked what had prevented them from registering. The two main reasons were hostile receptionists and needing a local address. One of the people interviewed in the report made this comment: 'When I said I was NFA to the receptionist, she said we're not taking any new patients on. I can tell when people don't like me' (Stern *et al.* 1989).

The study then asked those who had not attempted to register why they had not done so. The most frequent reason given by those sleeping rough was because they had thought there was no point. 'You can't register with a doctor if you're NFA' or 'No doctor in London will take you without an address.' Another group living in large hostels felt that registration was not a priority. Some felt that their mobility was a barrier. 'I move around a lot which is a problem for GPs. I haven't been to a doctor for a long time' (Stern *et al.* 1989). For others registration was a less urgent priority than finding a bed for the night or getting a hot meal.

Another reason cited as a barrier to access by some people was the offer of temporary registration. Commonly, homeless people perceive temporary registration as an avenue to a second-class service or as a polite way of saying 'we don't want people like you in this surgery'.

One man interviewed by a member of the East London Homeless Health Team, when asked what he would do if he felt unwell, gave the following reply:

Well there wasn't much that I could do. I would . . . try and shake it off . . . I did go to a doctor one day when I had chest trouble and I did ask whether he could take me on his books and he said no. Now whether that was the reason because he knew I was sleeping rough, because he asked me where I was living and I was honest with him and told him I was sleeping rough and he said No I can't take you on my books I'm full up at the moment, but he said I'll take you on

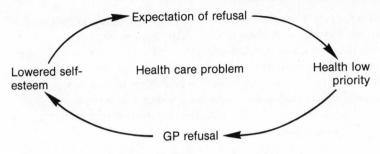

*Figure 2.1* The cycle of reluctance

temporary, I can't take you on as a full and I thought that may have been his polite way of telling me I don't want dossers on my book.

(Fisher 1989)

Access to primary health care is not governed solely by general practitioner reluctance nor are problems of access uniform across the homelessness spectrum. Both the West Lambeth study and that conducted by the PSI show that registering with a GP is not a priority for some homeless people. These studies also appear to indicate that the registration rates among those sleeping rough are particularly low and that here the barriers to access are almost unassailable. The unwillingness of GPs to register is compounded by the homeless person's expectation that they will be refused. This may in part be due to an accumulation of previous negative experiences by both parties. What emerges is a cycle of reluctance on the part of the GP and single homeless people. Added to this is the sense of powerlessness and stigmatization which inevitably has a corrosive effect on the individual's self-esteem.

The outcome of this cycle is that many homeless men and women who are sleeping rough or who have been homeless for long periods of time suffer from poor physical health which remains untreated until the disease process has reached an advanced state. See Figure 2.1.

Shiner, in his study of the health perception of single homeless people, *Adding Insult to Injury*, observed that apparent examples of 'apathy' can best be interpreted as rational judgements by people based on what they feel it is realistic to expect from their health given the conditions that they live in. Health expectations varied between those who were, or had been, sleeping on the streets and those who had not: while the former viewed ill health as the natural product of life on the streets, the latter were unprepared to make concessions regarding health on the basis of their homelessness. The notion of low health expectation helps to explain why some homeless people tend to seek health care only when illnesses have become serious.

Firsthand experiences are not the only influence on homeless people's attitudes to the various sources of care. Significant others influenced their behaviour, attitudes and expectations. It was on the advice of others that some people went straight to specialist providers and others knew which GP would register them if they were sleeping on the streets.

## Accident and emergency (casualty) access

Difficulties in obtaining access to primary health care services have meant that accident and emergency departments have been an important source of health care provision for some single homeless men and women. This is often considered to be a misuse of these facilities and questions are raised about their motivation: are they seeking treatment or a comfortable bed for the night?

> One thing which all casualty departments have in common . . . is the knowledge that virtually every homeless person needs a bed to sleep in. For this reason they are very concerned with the possibility of malingering and with the problems of accommodation which will confront the hospital on the patient's discharge.
>
> (Davies 1974)

Statistical estimates of the numbers of single homeless people attending accident and emergency departments have produced a confusing picture. This is not surprising, as any analysis requires a detailed knowledge of the hostels, squats, hotels, bed and breakfasts and other accommodation used by homeless people in the locality of the department. A number of estimates have however been made. Powell (1987) estimated that single homeless people in Edinburgh were five times more likely to use an accident and emergency department than were the housed population. He went on to argue that as many as 95 per cent of 'regular' attenders were single homeless people. In contrast, in an analysis of fourteen studies conducted between 1975 and 1984, SHIL (Single Homeless in London) found that the use of metropolitan accident and emergency departments by single homeless people averaged out at once daily per department. As SHIL commented, 'Homeless single people are among those who occasionally turn to Accident and Emergency Units for primary health care, but contrary to a generally held impression, such use is only occasional' (SHIL 1987).

The belief that homeless people who attend casualty departments are malingering has also been questioned. The West Lambeth study reported that three-quarters of the people they questioned who were sleeping out and had used accident and emergency departments listed injury or assault as their reason for using the service. Furthermore, a systematic analysis by Manchester CHC of the casualty records at three Manchester hospitals during a six-month period detected very few people who were not in need of treatment. For instance, 70.5 per cent of those presenting at the Manchester Royal Infirmary had exclusively casualty problems or required immediate admission compared with 28.5 per cent who were judged to be using the service inappropriately. The study concluded that 'abuse of casualty, far from being prevalent among homeless people, occurs only on a very small scale. The area to concentrate on is misuse – where homeless people do have genuine complaints but where often, through no fault of their own, they have come to the wrong place for treatment' (Manchester CHC 1980).

While the use of casualty departments by the single homeless may be statistically small and in the main for legitimate reasons, there is little doubt that they are still perceived as 'problem patients'; or, as one writer noted more graphically, 'It is the single homeless male with his stereotype dirty coat, with a bottle protruding from the pocket, who is the villain of the piece for the hospitals' (Thomas 1974). Ignorance and fear lie behind such attitudes which themselves are often based on a lack of training.

Discriminatory attitudes are also founded on a fear of violence or intimidation and on the feelings of powerlessness by already overworked and under-resourced staff. As City and Hackney CHC point out, 'It is not the fault of the staff that there is insufficient aftercare and housing provision. We must also understand the predicament of doctors who have few beds and have to make difficult decisions about those who can be admitted and those who can't' (Fowke *et al.* 1980).

The stereotype of the single homeless person as the 'lazy, crazy drunk' remains a powerful barrier to adequate accident and emergency treatment and gives rise to the occasional scandal. One such case which received national attention was that of Thomas Frazer, a 57-year-old man who died alone and untreated in a local graveyard after being turned away twice from a Hackney hospital because he was considered to be drunk. The post-mortem revealed that he had sustained a fractured skull and had died of a brain haemorrhage.

Casualty staff in inner cities have been slow to recognize the potential opportunity to intervene when unregistered (with a GP) homeless people do attend. Rarely in our experience are such people given a GP letter or directed to a known local GP or even the local FHSA to facilitate registration. Much locally based work is needed to improve this situation; central directives are unlikely to work, though, in areas where problems are prevalent, the FHSAs should consider having full-time representatives on site in casualty to help all unregistered attenders, homeless or not.

### In-patient provision and aftercare

With the exception of accident and emergency services and clinics for sexually transmitted disease, access to NHS hospital in-patient and out-patient services is achieved only by referral from a general practitioner.

This 'gatekeeper' role was in existence prior to the inception of the NHS, having evolved from the practical necessities occasioned by the facts that specialist consultant services are expensive and often at some distance from the patient, who may be unclear as to the exact nature of their problem or the specialist help available. The role was formalized in the NHS structure, first, to maximize the efficiency of hospital services in serving a 'screened' and therefore reduced population of patients and, second, to protect the position of general practitioners who feared that patients would, if able to do so at no direct cost, simply attend the hospital out-patient department of their choice.

This 'gatekeeping' function has many benefits and has been central to the success of the NHS in providing comprehensive care of high quality to all citizens at a cost affordable to the national purse.

For example:

- Patients are commonly seen, over time, by a GP whom they know, and who knows them, with different problems and episodes of illness.
- GPs can act as advocates and facilitators for patients in contact with hospital services.
- GPs can reflect the views and needs of patients through the NHS management structures – this has been especially important in the recent and current specification of contract service provision following the separation of purchaser/provider functions in the NHS reforms of 1991.
- Consultant specialists are focusing their attention on referred

patients who are considerably more likely to need and benefit from specialist intervention.

– More than 90 per cent of illness episodes are dealt with by GPs in the community. Such care is easily accessed, appropriately 'low technology' and very cost-effective.

While single homeless people make limited use of primary health care services they make far more extensive use of in-patient care than the general population. The West Lambeth study reported that, with the exception of people living in hostels, most sections of the homeless population used in-patient services two and half times as often as the general population. This suggests that this population has both a high incidence and a high tolerance of ill health and thus will seek treatment only when they are very ill.

While there is much evidence to the contrary, some studies have argued that high rates of in-patient admission are evidence that single homeless people are successfully manipulating admission via casualty departments into hospital beds. One article entitled 'Cost to the National Health Service of social outcasts with organic disease' by Drs Cooke and Grant was based on a single case study. This study argued that a

common misuse of NHS hospital facilities, for which the patients themselves are not wholly responsible, is made by patients, usually vagabonds or social outcasts, with a chronic or relapsing disease who gain admission to many different hospitals on numerous occasions. The admission is ostensibly for a treatment of the recurrence of the illness, but the patient's real motive may be to obtain a comfortable bed, nourishing meals, and other creature comforts when he is tired of sleeping rough or languishing in a lodging house.

(Cooke and Grant 1975: 132)

The study concluded:

Patients of the type we have described may number several thousands, and they must account for a sizeable proportion of NHS expenditure, particularly in the hospitals of our major cities and towns.

(Cooke and Grant 1975: 134)

Despite the colourful language and extravagant claims, Cooke and Grant inadvertently point to a problem which a number of studies have highlighted, namely aftercare. The majority of patients with a home and a caring family neither seek nor require early readmission to hospital.

For many single homeless patients discharge from hospital presents both problems and dangers, as they are forced to recuperate in unsuitable accommodation such as hostels or on the street. Many hostels are closed during the day and others will take patients directly from hospital only if some guarantee is offered of readmittance should it prove necessary. There are also a number of practical difficulties that the newly discharged homeless patient may have to face: toilet facilities may be situated several floors below or above, the accommodation they have been discharged to may not provide meals and for the less mobile stairs may prove difficult to negotiate. As Chatterton observes:

> Many hostels do not have the necessary facilities to provide aftercare and often only offer a return to a squalid, disease ridden environment to a patient new out of a warm supportive hospital environment. Access to appropriate aftercare support is limited.
>
> (Chatterton 1985)

In London there is a single ten-bedded aftercare facility where homeless people can convalesce. This does not take women and the number of beds is often reduced by direct admission from the project's Great Chapel Street Clinic.

The problem is further exacerbated by early discharge policies which are naturally built on the assumption that the patient has a roof over their head and carers available. Most homeless people by definition have neither of these. The cost of these policies to the well-being of many single homeless people who require in-patient admission together with the lack of appropriate aftercare is unknown. It requires little imagination to recognize that 'the resultant depression and social isolation may well lead to a downward spiral of ill health and increased depression, perhaps ending with relapse and further hospitalisation' (Fowke *et al.* 1980).

The most common reaction to these obstacles adopted by most single homeless people is to deny or minimize the importance of their own health problem or illness until it becomes overwhelming. This is in keeping with low self-esteem and poor perceptions of self-worth and becomes, given the constraints of their lifestyle, the best option for coping with a health problem in the short term.

# CONCLUSION

A commonly held belief is that single homeless people avoid the problem of access to GPs by simply using (or abusing) casualty departments. In fact this is not the case – single homeless people in urban areas are frequently seen at accident and emergency departments but analysis (Davison *et al.* 1983) shows that generally they are ill enough to warrant such attendances. Their lifestyle is often chaotic and actually traumatic, involving a much greater than average risk of accident, assault, wounds, burns, etc.

When/if their health problem becomes overwhelming homeless people will commonly (Davies 1974; Shiner 1991) seek help from agencies or workers outside the NHS as an avenue to care. Most often these are volunteer doctors/nurses working in charitable day/evening centres specifically aimed at the single homeless community and perceived by them to be accessible and less likely to be judgemental or rejecting in their approach. This marginalization is seen to be a bipartite process involving patient perceptions and illness behaviour as well as aspects of service provision and provider attitudes. These arguments are as true for housing and social care provision as for health care.

It follows from all this that single homeless people are more likely to present later in the development of an illness with more advanced disease than their housed contemporaries (Toon *et al.* 1987; John 1980) and that those homeless people suffering chronic illnesses, for example, epilepsy, diabetes, schizophrenia, are less likely to be able to receive personal and continuing care of optimum quality (John 1980).

We would agree that to minimize these various obstacles and improve access to, and quality of, care for single homeless people the NHS itself needs to adopt flexible and sensitive approaches to service provision for the single homeless community. Taking chiropody services as a simple example: the NHS does not provide chiropody services to adults under 65, except diabetics and pregnant women, yet foot problems and poor foot health are known to be very common among single homeless people, causing much discomfort and morbidity and some long-term disability. NHS chiropody services could be opened up to single homeless people and foot-care workers employed by health authorities and NHS trusts in areas with significant homeless populations. DSS footwear grants could be improved for NFA persons and hostel dwellers, a move which itself would prevent many foot health problems. These improvements could not be self-financing but would produce long-term savings through morbidity prevented. This example illustrates the basic elements of change required to make NHS services more accessible to single homeless people:

- Outreach work (foot-care workers) is often necessary in order to engage homeless people, especially street dwellers, and link them to available services while providing health education and raising their expectations. Novel roles, for example, nurse practitioners, may have an important part to play in developing 'outreach' activities.
- A flexible approach is required on the part of providers. Rigid exclusion criteria based on geography, age or diagnostic labels, foster inaccessibility and relaxations are a prerequisite if services to groups with demonstrable need are to improve. Such flexibility would produce gains in terms of morbidity prevented.
- Social needs as well as purely medical needs must be addressed (e.g. the provision of footwear). The two are inextricably linked and failure of health care provision to recognize and act to improve a patient's social well-being commonly leads to failure of treatment provided, failure to prevent future morbidity, failure to foster the concept of 'health as a priority' for the patient; and further loss of self-esteem. Added to this the likely success of future interventions is undermined.
- For any of these changes to be achieved requires a multidisciplinary, collaborative and integrated approach to health care provision at community level. This has never been successfully achieved by NHS provision to date.

## NOTE

1 Primary Care for Homeless People, Chalton Street, London NW1.

## REFERENCES

Acheson, D. (1981) 'Primary health care in inner London', *Report of a Study Group Commissioned by the London Health Planning Consortium*, London: DHSS.

Association of Community Health Councils in England and Wales/Campaign for Single Homeless People (1980) *Primary Care Provision for the Single Homeless. Findings of an ACHCEW/CHAR Survey*, ACHCEW/CHAR.

Association of General Practitioners in Urban Deprived Areas (1990) 'Report of Conference', AGUDA.

Brickner, P.W., Scanlan, B.C., Conanan, B., Elvy, A., MacAdam, J., Schare, L.K. and Vicnic, W.J. (1986) 'Homeless persons and health care', *Annals of Internal Medicine* 104: 405–9.

British Medical Association (1991) *Report to Council*, London: BMA.

Chatterton, C.S. (1985) *Homeless and Healthless*, unpublished BA thesis, University of London.

Cooke, N. and Grant, I.W.B. (1975) 'Cost to the National Health Service of social outcasts with organic disease', *British Medical Journal* 19(4): 132–4.

Crow, I., McDonough, O. and Roberts, S. (1977) *Primary Medical Care for the Homeless*, London: NACRO.

Davies, A. (1974) *Medical Care for Homeless and Rootless People*, London: CHAR.

Davison, A.G., Hildrey, A.C.C. and Floyer, M.A. (1983) 'The use and misuse of an accident and emergency department in the East End of London', *Journal of the Royal Society of Medicine* 5: 255–62.

Drake, M., O'Brien, M. and Biebuyck, C. (1982) *Single and Homeless*, London: HMSO.

Fisher, K. (1989) 'Interviews with day centre clients at St Botolph's Crypt Centre', unpublished.

Foster, P. (1983) *Access to Welfare*, London: Macmillan.

Fowke, B., Turner, T. and Coulter, P. (1980) *Homeless and Healthless*, London: City and Hackney Community Health Council.

Gaskell, P.G. (1969) 'Illnesses in lodging house inmates', *Health Bulletin* 1: 69.

Harrington, I. (1980) 'No place to call home', *Community Care* 12 October.

John, H.H. (1980) 'Primary care at hostels for alcoholics' *Health Trends* 12: 61–4.

Laidlaw, J. (1955) *Glasgow Common Lodging Houses and the People Living in Them*, Health and Welfare Committee, Glasgow Corporation.

Law, R. and Thompson, T. (1983) 'T.B. on the rise again in East End', *Observer* 10 April.

MacLean, D. and Newman, L. (1979) 'Primary care for the single homeless – the Edinburgh experiment', *Health Bulletin* 1: 79.

McCrory, M. (1975) *Sick and Homeless in the Grassmarket*, The Grassmarket Project.

Manchester Central Community Health Council (1980) *Health Care for Homeless People*, Manchester Central CHC.

*Mind News* (1980) 'High number of London's homeless mentally ill', July/ August.

No Fixed Abode (1974) 'Health and the Homeless in Tower Hamlets', NFA.

Powell, P.V. (1987) 'Use of accident and emergency departments by the single homeless', *Health Bulletin (Edinburgh)* 45(5): 255–62.

Ryan, W. (1971) *Blaming the Victim* , New York: Vintage Books.

Scott, R., Gaskell, P.G. and Morrell, D.C. (1966) 'Patients who reside in common lodging houses', *British Medical Journal*, 24(12): 1561–4.

SHIL (1987) 'Primary health care for homeless single people in London: a strategic approach', *Report of the Health Sub-group of the Joint Working Party on Single Homelessness in London*, London: SHIL.

Shiner, M. (1991) *Adding Insult to Injury*, unpublished Msc thesis, University of Surrey.

Stern , R., Stillwell, B. and Heuston, J. (1989) *From Margins to the Mainstream: Collaboration and Planning Services for Single Homeless People*, London: West Lambeth Health Authority, Priority Services Unit.

Taylor, C. (1987) 'Primary care in Liverpool' *Medicine in Society* 7.
Thomas, R. (1974) 'Where the last laugh may go to the villain of the piece', *Health Services Journal* 8 September.
Toon, P.D. (1985) 'Health and the homeless', *Christian Action Journal* spring.
Toon, P.D., Doherty, M. and Holden, H.M. (1975) 'Medical care for homeless and rootless young people', *British Medical Journal* 4: 446–8.
Toon, P.D., Thomas, K. and Doherty, M. (1987) 'Audit of work at a medical centre for the homeless over one year', *Journal of the Royal College of General Practitioners* 37: 102–22.
Williams, S. and Allen, I. (1989) *Healthcare for Single Homeless People*, London: PSI.

# 3 Health care for single homeless people

*John Balazs*

## INTRODUCTION

One of the difficulties faced by anyone trying to describe and analyse the health problems experienced by people who are single homeless is that they are not an homogeneous group. There are variations between different parts of the country as well as sub-populations of homeless people within specific areas. Homeless populations also change fairly rapidly, making accurate description difficult.

Furthermore, the aetiology of some of the health problems of homeless people is multifactorial and often very difficult to unravel. Some health problems may cause homelessness. A good example is chronic severe mental illness – in particular schizophrenia – where a person's ability to cope, the occurrence of relapse and the failure of appropriate therapy and community care can all combine to lead to a breakdown of a stable home environment and thus to homelessness. Some morbidity results from being homeless, for example, the high incidence of skin infestations (Committee on Health Care for Homeless People 1988: 45). Homelessness can also complicate and exacerbate pre-existing health problems. The treatment of leg ulcers, normally done in the community, may necessitate admission of a homeless person to a hospital or sick-bay to ensure thorough bedrest and good food.

The data used to illustrate this chapter come from the work of the East London Homeless Health Team (HHELP). The HHELP team provides an outreach primary care service to the single homeless in the East End of London. The outreach aspect is achieved by having surgeries in the places where many homeless people go. These places are mainly run by the voluntary sector and include a variety of day/evening centres, night-shelters, short- and longer-stay hostels and special units for homeless people with substance dependency problems. The team also sees patients on the streets. The general practitioners working with the team are all full-time local doctors with a special interest in caring for the homeless. All patients are encouraged to visit the general practitioners in their normal surgeries.

Most of the published work about the health problems of single homeless people has been based on hostel residents. A review by Powell (1988) outlines some of this material. To balance the bias towards the hostel-based population this chapter looks at the various sub-populations of the homeless in a number of different ways. The most important of these appear to be by age, sex, housing status and institution of first contact. It is thus possible to identify and describe the various sub-populations of homeless people in East London. Conclusions drawn from this work may be applied to homeless people in other parts of Britain.

## WHO ARE THE EAST END HOMELESS?

The HHELP team has seen 3,000 individuals over a four-year period. The team collects two types of information about these patients. One is a profile of the patient. This includes a full past medical history, sex, age, housing status – past and present, ethnic background, place of birth, marital and employment status, smoking, alcohol (in units per week) and a history of any regular drug use. Figure 3.1 shows the cumulative take-up of HHELP services over a four-year period.

The other type of data collected is a detailed analysis of each consultation or contact with any member of the team. This includes the nature of each presentation, i.e. why the patient has consulted, as viewed from the patient's perspective.

### Age

Until 1985 the population of single homeless people in the East End fitted the traditional stereotype. It was mainly made up of middle-aged white Caucasian men who lived, at least some of the time, in one of the local hostels. This group was fairly stable, most having been in the East End for several years (NFA 1986: 20). Surprisingly, the homeless appeared as stable as the housed population in East London, where there is up to a 30 per cent turnover per year (personal communication Alan Bennett, general manager, City & East London Family Health Services Authority).

In the last decade there have been very marked changes. First, the number of hostel spaces in the City and East London has declined from about 2,250 to under 500, a much sharper decline than in the rest

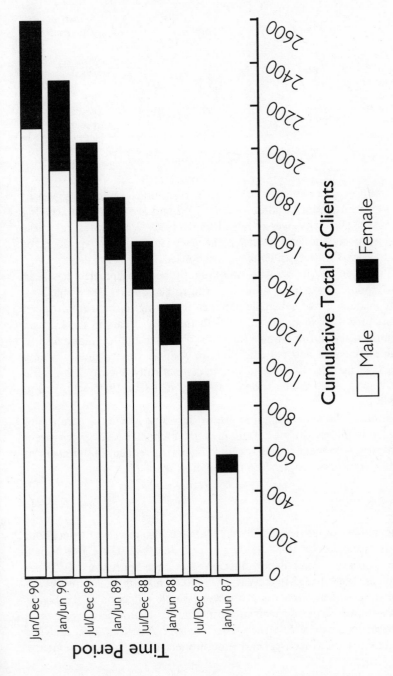

*Figure 3.1* Cumulative take-up of HHELP services (to December 1990)

*Table 3.1* Age range of all clients (men and women)

|  | 1987–9 | | 1990 | | Statistical |
|  | Total no. | % | Total no. | % | significance* |
|---|---|---|---|---|---|
| Under 20 | 52 | 2.6 | 48 | 8.5 | yes |
| 20 to 30 | 360 | 17.7 | 151 | 26.7 | yes |
| 31 to 40 | 470 | 23.1 | 155 | 27.4 | no |
| 41 to 50 | 535 | 26.3 | 124 | 21.9 | no |
| 51 to 60 | 359 | 17.7 | 59 | 10.4 | yes |
| 61 plus | 257 | 12.6 | 26 | 4.6 | yes |

*Source*: Smellie *et al.* 1991: 40.
*Note*: *chi squared using 1987–9 as expected numbers – significance at 0.01 level

of London. The reduction in the number of direct-access bedspaces in hostels throughout London between 1982 and 1987 was 7,200, leaving about 13,500 bedspaces (SHIL Report 1990: 21). Because of these energetic closure and resettlement programmes large numbers of middle-aged hostel residents were rehoused.

Provision for people who subsequently became homeless has been fairly poor. These 'new' homeless tend to be younger (see Table 3.1). The median age of new male patients presenting to the team dropped from forty-five years during 1988 to thirty-five years in the first six months of 1990. For women there was a similar, but less marked shift. The numbers of new patients who are younger women (under twenty years) in the year 1990 has increased dramatically. Figures 3.2 and 3.3 show the age/sex distribution for the period 1987 to 1989 inclusive and 1990.

Some of the underlying reasons for this rapid rise in the numbers of young homeless are described in a later chapter. However, recent central government initiatives have begun to reduce the numbers of young homeless people sleeping rough in the capital.

## Sex

The number of women seen by the team has also increased from about 14 per cent during 1988 to 22 per cent in 1990. There has been a concomitant increase in consultation rates from approximately 25 per cent in 1988 to 35 per cent in 1990. This higher frequency of consultation for women is probably a simple reflection of the higher consultation rates for women with primary health care workers in general (*Morbidity Statistics from General Practice* 1986: 23). The availability of women general practitioners has also recently greatly

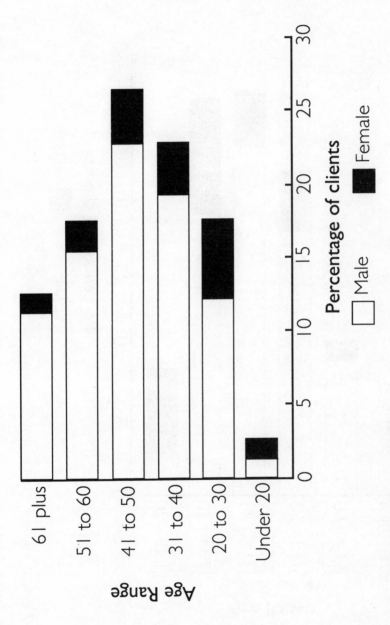

*Figure 3.2* Age range of clients (1987–9)

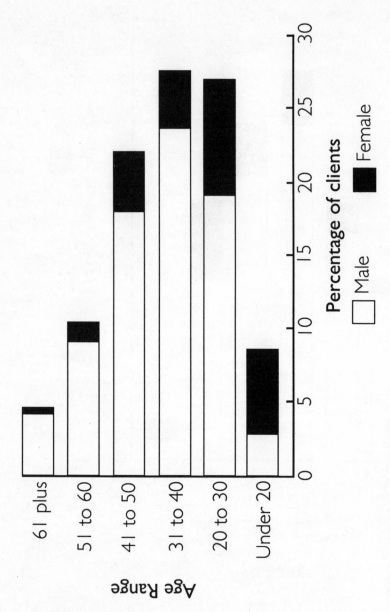

*Figure* 3.3 Age range of clients (1990)

increased. This may have contributed to the increased consultation rate because women doctors meet a previously unmet need. Another interesting point is the age distribution for women; they are predominantly young (see Figure 3.3).

## Ethnicity and place of birth

The majority (95 per cent) of people seen by the team were Caucasian. This might appear surprising given the ethnic breakdown of residents in parts of Tower Hamlets. Over 30 per cent of residents in Bethnal Green are Bangladeshi and yet less than 1 per cent of HHELP's patients were Bangladeshi. There are two main reasons why the team did not encounter homeless people from the ethnic minorities. First, the team works with the well-established voluntary sector (mainly church-based). These institutions did not cater for the needs of the ethnic minorities and therefore did not attract clients from non-Caucasian ethnic backgrounds. Second, homelessness among Bangladeshis is expressed in the form of poor housing and severe overcrowding rather than rooflessness (Richards 1989: 13).

The place of birth of HHELP's patients (Figure 3.4) reflects their ethnic background. There appear to have been no significant changes between 1987 and 1990.

Table 3.2 gives a breakdown of the 5 per cent of HHELP's patients from the ethnic minorities.

## Accommodation

In Table 3.3 there is a breakdown of the accommodation status on first contact with the team for patients over a four year period. Over the last year there has been a relative increase in the numbers of clients seen by the team who live on the streets or in temporary accommodation (62 per cent to 71 per cent) and a decrease in the numbers living in secure accommodation (38 per cent to 30 per cent). Fewer people from longer-stay hostels were seen by the team because of the reduction in bedspaces and the closure of a number of these institutions. The percentage of people living in stable accommodation is a reflection of the resettlement work done in East London which made these closures possible. Clients often continue to use both the services of the team and the voluntary sector after they have been resettled. Of the 3,000 clients seen less than 2 per cent were living in private rented accommodation, a reflection of the massive decline in this form of tenure.

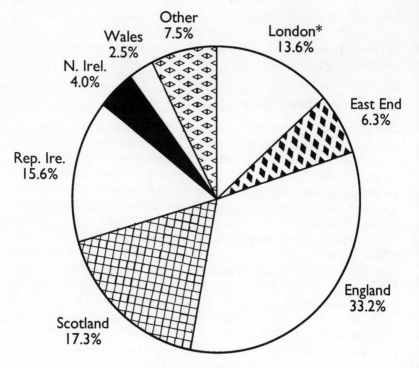

Figure 3.4 Place of birth of clients (1987–90)

Table 3.2 Ethnic breakdown of HHELP clients

| Ethnic group | 1987–90 | |
| | Number | Percentage |
| --- | --- | --- |
| West Indian | 44 | 33.8 |
| Asian | 33 | 25.3 |
| African | 31 | 23.8 |
| Other | 21 | 16.2 |
| Total | 129 | |

*Source*: Smellie *et al.* 1991: 40.

*Table 3.3* Accommodation status of new clients

| Accommodation | 1987–9 | | 1990 | |
| --- | --- | --- | --- | --- |
| | Number | Percentage | Number | Percentage |
| NFA/street | 577 | 28.4 | 169 | 31.9 |
| Short-stay hostel | 473 | 23.3 | 131 | 24.8 |
| Long-stay hostel | 405 | 19.9 | 88 | 16.6 |
| Council | 275 | 13.5 | 47 | 8.4 |
| Squat | 74 | 3.6 | 22 | 4.2 |
| Hotel/B & B | 41 | 2.0 | 11 | 2.1 |
| Friends | 37 | 1.8 | 14 | 2.6 |
| Private rented | 29 | 1.4 | 8 | 1.4 |
| Special unit | 14 | 0.7 | 20 | 3.8 |
| Housing association | 23 | 1.1 | 3 | 0.6 |
| Owner-occupier | 18 | 0.9 | 1 | 0.2 |
| Family | 7 | 0.3 | 7 | 1.3 |
| Resettlement unit | 14 | 0.7 | 0 | |
| Not recorded | 35 | 1.7 | 36 | 6.4 |

*Source*: Smellie *et al.* 1991: 41.

*Table 3.4* HHELP patients – accommodation status of those seen only once by GPs in 1991

| Type of accommodation | Number* |
| --- | --- |
| NFA | 142 |
| Unstable | 130 |
| Stable | 42 |
| Total | 314 |

*Note*: *data collected for the first ten months of 1991.

HHELP's clients are fairly mobile. In 1989 48 per cent of patients on the first and subsequent consultations had been in their particular accommodation or NFA for a month or less. However, the majority of those seen by the team appeared to have strong roots in the East End. Individuals who were sleeping on the streets were more likely to be seen once only (see Table 3.4) which highlights one of the major difficulties of providing continuity of care to this group of patients.

There were significant shifts of clients within various forms of unstable accommodation and between unstable accommodation and NFA. The shift into stable accommodation from other groups is low. Table 3.5 details these movements in accommodation sub-groups in

*Table 3.5* HHELP patients – shift between different types of accommodation in 1991

| Accommodation at first contact 1991 | Accommodation at last contact in 1991 | | | |
|---|---|---|---|---|
| | NFA | Unstable | Stable | Total |
| NFA | 72 | 32 | 8 | 112 |
| unstable | 14 | 118 | 12 | 144 |
| stable | 1 | 6 | 70 | 77 |
| total | | | | 333 |

*Table 3.6* Changes in accommodation status of one 38-year-old man who had regular contact with two different HHELP GPs in 1991*

| Date of contact | Accommodation status |
|---|---|
| 10 January | NFA |
| 31 January | NFA |
| 7 February | NFA |
| 11 February | NFA |
| 11 March | NFA |
| 21 March | squat |
| 18 April | squat |
| 16 May | NFA |
| 30 May | NFA |
| 22 June | squat |
| 8 July | NFA |
| 15 July | short-stay hostel |
| 22 July onward | NFA |

*Note*: *he stayed in East London throughout this time.

the first ten months of 1991 among patients seen, on at least two occasions, by HHELP general practitioners.

While this table gives only a crude impression of mobility, a more detailed analysis of one patient's movements is contained in Table 3.6. He started and ended the study period on the streets.

**Registration with general practitioners**

One of the aims of the HHELP team is to facilitate the registration of homeless people with general practitioners. Of all the patients seen, 40 per cent had general practitioners in London (Smellie *et al.* 1991: 42). Three-quarters of these doctors worked in the East End. Most of these registered patients were living in secure accommodation. However, 76 per cent of patients in insecure accommodation (including NFA) were

not registered, whereas only 23 per cent of those in secure accommodation were not registered. Most homeless people encountered by
HHELP were therefore not registered with a general practitioner.

Thirty-seven per cent of all HHELP's patients did try to register
with general practitioners in the year prior to contact with the team.
The majority of these people succeeded in registering (77 per cent were
taken onto a general practitioner's list and 23 per cent were refused).
This is a slightly higher registration rate than in other parts of London
(Stern *et al.* 1988: appendix K). Many clients were reluctant to register
with general practitioners in East London, even though many of the
barriers to registration no longer exist.

About 70 per cent of patients had, on first contact with the team, no
recent contact with other health care workers. This, taken with the
relatively poor general practitioner registration, is a strong argument
in favour of an outreach primary health care service.

Registration with a general practitioner ensures that a homeless
person receives the same quality of service as a housed person. An
argument frequently put forward supporting the aim of registration
with a general practitioner is that of gaining information from the
patients' previous medical records; in Britain these follow patients
each time they register with a new doctor (Single Homeless in London
1990: 21).

The author carried out a survey comparing the information obtained by HHELP from the patient and other sources with that obtained
from the patient's definitive notes from the Family Practitioner
Committee (now called the FHSA). *None* of the 100 FPC notes
contained information not already available to HHELP. Many of the
FPC notes were hopelessly out of date, as the patients had not been
registered with a GP for a number of years. Most were disorganized, a
problem of GP notes in general, especially in the inner cities. In
addition the mobility of some homeless patients often means their
notes will never catch up with their current GP.

All patients who see a HHELP general practitioner register with
that doctor. Thus the aim of integrating homeless people into ordinary
mainstream services is achieved. Many of the patients now consult
their general practitioners in their ordinary surgeries rather than in the
voluntary sector institution where they first made contact.

## WHY DO HOMELESS PEOPLE CONSULT WITH GPs?

Analysis of HHELP's data shows that many homeless people present
to health care workers with a spectrum of problems similar to those of

*Table 3.7* Comparison of observed and expected number of consultations for each disease group

| Disease group | Expected | Percentage*<br>Found in 1990 | Statistical<br>significance** |
|---|---|---|---|
| Respiratory | 21.8 | 17.4 | no |
| Cardiovascular | 11.9 | 4.2 | yes |
| Gastrointestinal | 8.8 | 9.9 | no |
| Musculoskeletal | 11.6 | 20.1 | yes |
| Dermatological | 5.7 | 21.8 | yes |
| Mental health | 10.5 | 32.7 | yes |
| Nervous system | 6.2 | 4.3 | no |
| Trauma | 8.9 | 9.1 | no |
| Social/other | 6.9 | 42.9 | yes |
| Alcohol-related⁺ | – | 19.2 | – |
| Drug abuse⁺ | – | 10.4 | – |

*Notes*: *2,200 consultations altogether;
** significance at 0.1 level (chi test used);
⁺ other work indicates these are higher than expected (see Tables 3.11; 3.12; 3.13).
*Sources*: Smellie *et al.* 1991: 24
*Morbidity Statistics for General Practice* 1982: 62–101.

housed people. Overall, however, there are significant differences from what would have been expected from matched housed patients. Table 3.7 compares the reasons why homeless people presented to the HHELP general practitioners in 1990 as compared with, social-class-matched, expected presentation (*Morbidity Statistics for General Practice*, 1982: 102–13).

These comparisons are however much over-simplified. There are a number of factors which make detailed analysis very difficult. Although presentations may appear similar, the underlying pathology may be different. A number of examples appear later in this chapter.

HHELP's findings are similar to those of Shanks (1988), who analysed consultation data from his work in Manchester between July 1979 and December 1982. After matching for social class, the morbidity for homeless and for housed patients is very different. He found that the number of homeless people consulting with some conditions was much less than expected. He concluded:

High consultation rates in some groups (psychiatric and dermatological conditions) were balanced by low consultation rates in other groups. Thus the provision (of work load) to the homeless is

*Table 3.8* Consultation rates for male and female patients with a male and a female doctor at the Providence Row hostel* between January 1990 and September 1991

| Sex of patients | Male doctor | Female doctor | Statistical significance** |
|---|---|---|---|
| Male | 134 (44.2%) | 153 (36.3%) | yes |
| Female | 169 (55.8%) | 268 (63.7%) | yes |

*Notes:* *a mixed short-stay hostel;
**using chi squared test with consultations of female doctor as expected – significance > than 0.05 level.

shown to be no greater than to the general population, after adjustment for social class.

(Shanks 1988)

However, the HHELP Team would disagree with his conclusion, as the mix of medical and social problems found among the homeless imposes more work on the primary health care team than do housed patients.

If a similar group of patients have a choice of general practitioners they will often select one doctor in preference to another for specific problems. There are considerable differences in the consulting patterns of the HHELP general practitioners. One example of this is the preference women have for seeing a woman doctor. Table 3.8 compares the presenting complaints to two doctors – a man and a woman – working in the same mixed hostel on alternate weeks. These differences were statistically significant. The HHELP general practitioners include several women doctors and in 1990 they were responsible for over half of all consultations.

Each of the institutions in East London also has its own character. They cater for different groups and attract different homeless clients. For instance, the health care problems of men in a long-stay hostel are radically different from those of women attending a day centre on a women-only day or the residents of a short-stay direct-access hostel, mainly young people.

The outcomes of consultations with HHELP general practitioners in 1990 are also detailed in Figure 3.5. These outcomes reflect the variety of presenting problems, underlying disease, addiction, social and accommodation problems the homeless have. Interestingly, over half of all consultations involved advice or just a chat. Many homeless people value the opportunity to talk in an ordinary manner to a sympathetic person. While there is often very little traditional medical content to these consultations, they are extremely valuable for the patients, if only because they know there are people who will listen to them in a nonjudgemental way.

Thirteen per cent of all consultations had some preventive element.

## HEALTH PROBLEMS

I went to one hospital in London when I had pneumonia. There was a Canadian doctor there. He wasn't much interested in treating me once I had told him I was No Fixed Abode – the three magic words. He showed me across the road which was Mortimer Street and there were all these cardboard boxes and go and join them. I mean that's a nice way to treat homeless people, but then again I suppose it's because we're homeless.

(Pat Daley in *A Nice Way to Treat People* 1987: 2)

This comment illustrates a number of points, not least the disappointing attitude of some health professionals and the low health expectations of many people sleeping on the streets. However, treating someone who is homeless, with an acute medical condition such as pneumonia, can be problematic. In general practice most patients with a chest infection are treated at home with antibiotics and are usually nursed by relatives. This is not possible for someone who is homeless. Indeed, treating a homeless person often necessitates a 'social admission'.

In a recent review of the utilization of acute hospital services in London by homeless people, Shever *et al.* (1991) found that the cost of an unplanned admission to hospital for some homeless people was significantly greater than the cost of admission to more secure accommodation. Homeless patients also spent a longer time in hospital than other patients. This may partly explain the negative attitude of some hospital doctors to the homeless. The 'bed blocker' is never very popular, especially in the present climate when the pressure on beds in most hospitals is severe.

What is evident is that the extra cost of hospital care for homeless people has resource implications. These need to be taken into account by Regional Health Authorities when they allocate money for purchasing services in areas with large numbers of homeless people.

Non-compliance may also be problematic. A small audit on number of prescriptions actually dispensed was undertaken by the author in one quarter of 1988. Less than 40 per cent were actually dispensed (this

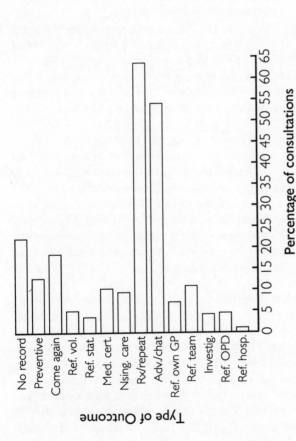

*Figure 3.5* Outcomes of consultations with general practitioners (1990)

*Note:* abbreviations used
ref. vol. – refer to voluntary sector
ref. stat. – refer statutory sector
med. cert. – medical certificate
nsing. care – refer to a nurse
Rx/repeat – prescription or repeat prescription or treatment

adv./chat – advice or chat
ref. own GP – patient referred back to their own GP
investig. – investigation, e.g. blood test or X-ray
ref. OPD – refer to out-patients department
ref. hosp. – refer to hospital for in-patient care

was for all groups of drugs not just antibiotics). This understandably has significant consequences for compliance with therapy. To overcome this problem, the HHELP team increased the proportion of drugs dispensed directly to its patients.

The rest of this chapter concentrates on some of the health issues which are of particular importance to the single homeless.

## Respiratory problems

Throughout the period of HHELP's work, the percentage of consultations where a respiratory problem was the main complaint has remained the same at around 17 per cent. The incidence in ordinary general practice is similar. However, there are significant differences in the types of respiratory problems the homeless have. The incidence of lower, as opposed to upper, respiratory tract is higher. An analysis of patients presenting to the HHELP team with respiratory problems in 1989 illustrates this. This is a very different pattern from that of the housed population where upper respiratory tract infections predominate (*Morbidity Statistics for General Practice* 1986: 96–7). Lower respiratory tract infections are less likely to resolve spontaneously, are more likely to need antibiotics and take longer to settle.

The reasons for this are multifactorial. No good research has been carried out with homeless people to elucidate the causes. One can merely try to extrapolate from work done with housed patients. Poor nutritional status has a part to play. Institutional settings, in either hostels or day centres, facilitate the spread of infections (Connelly *et al.* 1991: 67). This is especially true for influenza and tuberculosis. Damp environments have been shown to increase the incidence and severity of chronic respiratory problems (Martin and Platt 1987). Cold conditions lead to an excess mortality and morbidity (Curwen and Davis 1988).

Smoking is much commoner among homeless people. At least 85 per cent of men (sample size 2,077) and 76 per cent (sample size 496) of women encountered by HHELP smoked, whereas the prevalence of smoking in social class 5 is 43 per cent for men and 39 per cent for women (*Social Trends* 1991: 121). Tackling smoking is very difficult. Smoking is one of the major underlying causes of the increased respiratory morbidity among the single homeless. Featherstone and Ashmore (1988) conducted a small survey which found that over 40 per cent of the residents of a men's hostel suffered with chronic bronchitis. However, as one of our own patients pointed out, 'smoking's the only joy I have . . . and now you want to take it away from me'. Having no smoking areas in hostels may be a start. When this was raised at one of the hostels in East London, it was opposed on the grounds that it may 'drive the homeless away'. Personal counselling from a general practitioner or a nurse may have more of an effect. This is certainly true for housed clients, therefore why not for homeless people?

Excessive use of alcohol also has a significant part to play. A Canadian study (Schmidt and de Lint 1969) showed that death rates from pneumonia were three times greater in alcoholic men and seven times greater in alcoholic women than in the general population. Alcohol abuse is a major problem among homeless people in East London.

Housed patients can call on the support of families and friends when they, for example, have a chest infection, enabling them to be cared for at home. Homeless people cannot. For homeless people access to either special sick-bays, such as Wytham Hall (1990) in West London, or special beds in some hostels, such as resettlement units with their own nurses, may be the answer during the acute stages of a potentially fatal but usually curable illness such as pneumonia.

**Tuberculosis**

Tuberculosis (TB) has been a controversial area. In the past the prevalence of TB among hostel residents has been high; however, the relationship between TB and homelessness is a complex one. In England and Wales there has been a dramatic decline in the incidence of tuberculosis in all groups other than new immigrants from the Third World. In South Central London the incidence of TB declined from 1.3 per 1,000 in 1955 to 0.2 per 1,000 in 1986 (Stevens *et al.* 1991). This latter figure is three times above the average for England and Wales. About 7 per cent of these notifications (i.e. thirty-five individuals) were hostel residents. Very recently (1988–9) there appears to have been a slight increase in the incidence of TB in South London. As yet it is unclear why this has happened.

Since the Second World War mobile mass X-ray screening has been used to pick up new cases of TB in hostel-based populations. An editorial in the *Lancet* ('Tuberculosis and the alcoholic', 1979) concluded:

the homeless alcoholic represents a substantial pool of tuberculous infection. Mass X-ray screening . . . would lead to earlier diagnosis in this vulnerable group. Such efforts will be wasted unless they can be backed up by treatment which includes some social rehabilitation or social care.

Things have changed dramatically in the last decade. In South London the yield of new cases of tuberculosis was so low that the mass mobile X-ray service was discontinued in 1989. In a prospective study (Stevens *et al.* 1991) from 1985–7 547 single homeless hostel residents were screened using the mass miniature mobile X-ray. No new cases of TB were found. Two patients did have evidence of TB; however, both were already known and were under treatment. The screening did, on the other hand, pick up a few other clinical problems.

HHELP's work in East London paints a slightly different picture, probably because the population included the street homeless, not just the hostel based. In the two years 1988–90 thirteen cases of active tuberculosis were picked up. All except one had a serious drinking problem. Ten were reactivations of old tuberculosis. Seven of the cases were picked up in the Salvation Army alcohol detoxification unit among men who had previously been sleeping on the streets (all these men had their chest X-rays at the local hospital not the mass X-ray service). Another two patients were sleeping rough at the time of their X-rays. One man, the only one in stable accommodation, was immunosuppressed because he also had leukaemia and a drink problem. All the cases were picked up by either the doctors or the nurse specialists on clinical grounds. Some of these patients had their initial chest X-rays at a mobile mass X-ray site which offered much easier access to homeless clients than the local hospitals (one of which runs an appointments system). The last four years of mass X-ray in East London aimed at the single homeless revealed only three cases of tuberculosis among the homeless. The total number X-rayed was 1,182 (unpublished data, North East Thames mass X-ray screening service).

These findings concur with those of Ramsden *et al.* (1988). In a retrospective study carried out in West London they identified only nineteen cases out of 6,224 new patients seen in 1984–8. All these cases were detected clinically, none through mass X-ray screening. Fourteen of these patients abused alcohol. Ramsden *et al.*'s study also highlighted difficulties in compliance with drug treatment, with only one-third of their patients achieving a cure after one year. They proposed a number of reasons why this might be: alcohol abuse, suspicion of authority and probably a lack of appropriate shelter being the foremost of these. They concluded that the existence of special 'sick-bays' such as Caplin House in East London and Wytham Hall in

West London where homeless people with tuberculosis could stay until treatment was well established and alternative shelter was found may improve the cure rates of TB.

The fear that homeless people act as a reservoir of TB is probably no longer justified, certainly in relation to the general population. On a practical level, the people most at risk are the staff of voluntary sector and health care workers who come into daily contact with the single homeless. In East London two hostel workers contracted TB in 1987–9 and there were no policies for the screening of staff in a number of the centres. With the help of a chest physician at the London Chest Hospital a protocol was devised for the control of TB among the staff working with the single homeless in East London (see Appendix 3). This was based on recent advice from the British Thoracic Society (Skinner *et al.* 1990) on the control of TB in NHS employees.

**Mental health**

> not just my health but my nerves. You become like a bag of nerves. You're not settled, you're afraid all the time. You don't sleep properly unless you're really exhausted, you know, through roaming about all day. Your feet ache. Your whole body aches.
>
> (Phil aged forty, homeless for ten years,
> on the effects of sleeping rough on his health)

The comment above illustrates one extremely important point: most homeless people are very depressed at being homeless. Indeed, depression is a 'normal' reaction to being homeless. When consulting with homeless people it is all too easy to became oblivious to this depression. However, this is not to say that it is unimportant. The depression may act to reinforce someone's feelings of powerlessness, may contribute to poor motivation and encourage abuse of alcohol and minor tranquillizers.

Trying to unravel any possible aetiological links between homelessness and mental ill-health is extremely difficult. There is a lot of evidence that the causes of psychiatric disorders are multifactorial. While there is a wider discussion concerning causation in a later chapter, two of the less obvious factors to mention here are overcrowding (especially in day centres and hostels) and a lack of personal 'defensible space' (Mitchell 1976: 297).

Most of the published work about mental illness and homelessness concentrates on chronic psychosis (i.e., schizophrenia, manic and 'psychotic' depression) affecting hostel dwellers. There has been very little work on the true prevalence of severe chronic mental illness among the street homeless. The government has made considerable sums of money available through its 'Homeless Mentally Ill Initiative' on the assumption that the prevalence of mental illness is similar in different sub-populations of the homeless.

The assumption that there are large numbers of severely disturbed psychiatric 'patients' on the streets may not actually be the case. HHELP's work in East London illustrates this (Rapley *et al.* 1991). A patient was labelled as having chronic psychosis only if that patient fulfilled International Classification of Disease criteria. Each patient's diagnostic label was regularly reviewed if they continued to be in contact with the team. Without doubt the HHELP team under-estimated the prevalence of severe mental illness as team members were not able to take full psychiatric histories from most of the patients. However, patients were not labelled as schizophrenic on the basis of a brief consultation. Weller *et al.*'s report (1987) on 'Crisis at Christmas' suggested that thirty-four clients out of one hundred were 'actively psychotic'. How do such misinterpretations arise? Roth *et al.* concluded that:

> Traditional interpretations about symptomatology were confused by the fact that a homeless lifestyle typically includes characteristics and behaviours that can be the result of either mental illness or the stresses of street life, or both . . . the most prevalent items describing a dirty and dishevelled appearance and a flattened affect. While these may be signs of mental illness, they most surely can be the result of the exigencies of a homeless life style.
>
> (Roth *et al.* 1986: 313)

The author reviewed sixty-one patients seen by the HHELP team with a definite chronic mental health problem over one year in 1988–9. Half these patients were resident in long-stay hostels and the other half were either NFA or living in temporary accommodation. Forty-three of these had a diagnosis of schizophrenia, eight had affective disorders (bipolar and major depressive disorders). Ten patients had a variety of diagnostic labels (bulimia, psychopathic personality disorder and chronic alcoholic hallucinosis). Only ten had a past history of drug abuse and eleven gave a history of alcohol abuse. Fifty-one patients (84 per cent) had been admitted to a psychiatric hospital in the past.

On follow-up the diagnoses of three patients initially labelled as schizophrenic were changed: two to alcoholic hallucinosis and one to psychopathic personality disorder. Probably the diagnoses of more

*Table 3.9* Accommodation status among schizophrenics*

| Type of accommodation | Number (equals percentage) |
|---|---|
| Hostel short-stay | 32 |
| Hostel long-stay | 27 |
| NFA | 21 |
| Night-shelter | 9 |
| Council | 5 |
| Hotel/B & B | 2 |
| Squat | 1 |
| Housing association | 1 |
| Family | 1 |
| Resettlement unit | 1 |

*Note*: *seen by HHELP team in the four years until October 1991

patients would have been changed had contact been maintained with more patients over a longer period.

Only two-thirds of the patients returned for follow-up. This underlines one of the main problems in looking after the homeless mentally ill – the difficulty of providing continuing care. Sixty-two per cent of these patients were receiving medication. This is higher than in Phil Timms's study (Timms 1989: 70). This may be explained by the prior existence of easily accessible primary care services for these patients.

Between 1987 and 1991 the HHELP team has encountered one hundred individuals with schizophrenia. Almost half were women (forty-seven). In Table 3.9 there is a breakdown of their accommodation status at the time of first contact with the team. Most were in wholly inappropriate accommodation.

HHELP's work with homeless women who suffered from severe mental health problems really confirms the work of others. The prevalence of these problems appears to be about three times higher than in the men. The women seemed to be more severely disordered. There are number of reasons why this might be the case – all of them speculative. A woman may find it easier to stay within her family and remain in some sort of shelter than a man. For a woman to become homeless she may well be more disturbed, socially isolated and/or chaotic. These women are more vulnerable than homeless men and yet the HHELP team found making contact and maintaining ongoing relationships with them more difficult. This is another area where more research needs to be done.

The HHELP team's interventions with those patients with whom contact was maintained is interesting. Most of those in long-stay hostels remained in the same accommodation at the end of one year. Overall there was no change in the drug treatment status of these patients. (This is a situation which may improve with the advent of the 'Homeless Mentally Ill Initiative'.)

This contrasts with those in temporary accommodation or on the streets. Ten of these patients were moved into more secure accommodation. This included specialist units for the mentally ill, long-stay hostels and bed & breakfast. Two patients were readmitted to long-stay psychiatric hospitals (one in Glasgow and one in Leicester). One woman returned home to South America (again with help from HHELP). Two patients were admitted to psychiatric hospital because they were acutely ill. The HHELP team's involvement was crucial. The successful interventions were the initiation of counselling and drug therapy where appropriate and sorting out accommodation. This latter intervention often involved referral to the local authority homeless persons' unit and led to a dramatic improvement in that individual's quality of life. The two key workers in this process were the community psychiatric nurse and the social worker.

The difference in accommodation outcome between long-stay hostel dwellers and other homeless people is worrying. One possible explanation may be a degree of complacency on the part of carers when dealing with someone with a mental health problem who has been in a long-stay hostel for a while. There is also the problem of a lack of appropriate placement following long-term institutionalization in a hostel. With a person on the streets or in a short-stay hostel the problem of better accommodation is more obviously pressing. Perhaps more energy is expended by health care and social workers in improving a client's accommodation under these circumstances.

The difficulty of providing continuing care to people who are homeless and mentally ill is discussed in more detail in a later chapter. One possible way of overcoming some of these problems is to give the patients their own records to carry around. The author and Dr Reuler (1991) piloted such a patient-held record for the chronically mentally ill. Although a quarter of the records were lost or stolen over an eighteen-month period it was concluded that a patient-held medical record is feasible for homeless individuals. These records are also useful to other carers in providing a certain amount of basic information and a contact for possible co-ordination of care. All except one of the patients found pleasure in reading their medical records.

Easy access to mainstream psychiatric services is very important from a general practitioner's point of view. The barriers formed by strict adherence to catchment areas are formidable. The case of one patient cared for by HHELP illustrates this. A very disturbed acutely psychotic paranoid middle-aged schizophrenic man agreed to be admitted to hospital for his own safety. He was refusing to eat because he believed all his food was poisoned. He had left his home town in Scotland because of these paranoid ideas. HHELP contacted five local psychiatric hospitals as it was felt he needed admission. They all declined: two on the grounds that he was actually not their responsibility but the responsibility of his own health board in Scotland; one because they would take someone from out of the catchment area only if the patient was under section (not possible in this case as he was willing to go to hospital voluntarily!); the two others on the grounds of not having any acute male psychiatric beds. Eventually he was repatriated to his home town. This involved arranging a flight to take him back to Scotland. He remained on the streets until this was done as he was too fearful to go to a hostel.

A very worrying recent development is the refusal of some psychiatrists in inner London to see homeless patients, even those known to them previously, on the grounds that there are now psychiatric services specifically for homeless people. This actually increases the marginalization of homeless mentally ill men and women – the exact opposite of what recent initiatives for the homeless mentally ill were meant to achieve.

## Skin problems

These accounted for almost 22 per cent of all consultations with HHELP general practitioners in 1990. This is significantly more than would have been expected for a social class matched population (see Table 3.7, p. 62). Infestations with scabies and lice and other skin infections accounted for over a third of all skin problems encountered in 1989. This is much higher than would have been expected for the housed population (*Morbidity Statistics from General Practice* 1986: 145, 163). Some of these infestations were complicated by secondary, mainly pustular, infection. Successful treatment requires access to clothes' washing facilities and bathing facilities, as well as the careful application of anti-insect medication. The best time to do this is at the time of diagnosis.

Problems stemming from poor circulation to the legs are the other main group of skin problems which affect homeless people. The reasons why this should be are unclear and require further research. Spending a lot of time walking or standing, poor nutrition and limited access to regular washing facilities all may have a part to play. Leg

*Table 3.10* Temperature and morbidity

| Temperature (centigrade) | |
| --- | --- |
| 21°C | Room temperature recommended by the British Geriatrics Society in the winter of 1988 |
| 18°C | Comfortable level for most people |
| 16°C | Respiratory problems become more common |
| 12°C | Cardiovascular changes increase the risk of heart attack and stroke |
| 5°C | Significant increase in the risk of hypothermia |

*Source*: Lowry 1991: 16.

ulcers, varicose veins and varicose eczema are the commonest present-ations. Treatment involves nursing care, access to washing facilities, antibiotics for secondary infections and for the more obstinate cases access to shelter and bed-rest. This is especially true of leg ulcers, where an admission to an institution where nursing care is available may be the only short-term cure.

**Cold**

Low temperature is an important cause of morbidity and mortality among the homeless. In Britain for each degree Celsius that the winter is colder than average there are an extra 8,000 deaths. Most of these deaths are from respiratory (Curwen and Davis 1988) and cardio-vascular disease (Bull and Morton 1978). Table 3.10 summarizes the relation between temperature and some health changes (Lowry 1991: 16). Since homeless people are literally 'out in the cold', they are likely to suffer excess morbidity as the temperature drops.

Hypothermia does still occur. It usually happens where there is some other pre-existing medical problem, such as alcoholism, and is commoner in older patients. However, the incidence of diseases related to severe cold, such as frost-bite, is very low. HHELP encountered only two cases of frost-bite over the four-year study period. This can be explained by the relatively mild winters over this period and increased vigilance among the carers of the homeless. Organizations such as CRISIS not only provide warm shelter at the coldest time of year but also highlight the importance of keeping warm.

Table 3.11 Alcohol consumption among homeless women in East London v. United Kingdom expected (all social classes)

| Amount drunk[+] | Homeless women | | Expected* | Statistical significance[++] |
|---|---|---|---|---|
| None | 210 | 43.3% | 10% | yes |
| Occasional | 137 | 28.5% | 82% | yes |
| Moderate | 34 | 7.0% | 6% | no |
| Problem | 28 | 5.8% | 1% | yes |
| Harmful | 76 | 15.7% | 1%** | yes |
| | 485*** | | | |

Source: *Goddard 1991: 26
[+]Table B (ibid.)
Notes: **according to Goddard (1991: 31) the percentage of harmful drinking is 3% in unskilled manual women (i.e. social class V) – this is also statistically significant;
[++]chi squared at 0.05 significance level;
***HHELP data between early 1987 and June 1991.

## Alcohol

Alcohol misuse is unfortunately common among homeless people in East London. This section will concentrate on the medical consequences of these problems as other aspects are covered in a later chapter.

HHELP quantified alcohol consumption among its patients in units per week (see Appendix B). There were marked differences between various sub-groups of homeless people. People living on the streets tended to drink more than those in temporary or more permanent accommodation. Other important determining factors included sex and age; these are detailed in Tables 3.11 and 3.12. It is apparent that the incidence of alcohol problems among homeless women is much lower than among men. This is changing as younger homeless women in East London drink more than their older peers, which follows the national pattern (Goddard 1991: 27). More research needs to be done into why homeless women behave differently from men.

Almost half of the men (sample size 2,101) seen by HHELP drank harmful amounts of alcohol. Superficially this seems to fit in with the stereotype of the homeless alcoholic. However, these figures are skewed because the HHELP GPs looked after a male alcohol detoxification unit, where they saw two hundred and twenty-four men (though most of these men were homeless).

Contact making is the first step in helping a homeless person with a drink problem. This can be done by any easily accessible primary health care worker or specialist service such as a 'shop-front'. The next

*Table 3.12* Alcohol consumption among homeless men in East London v. United Kingdom expected (all social classes)

| Amount drunk⁺ | Homeless men | | Expected* | Statistical significance⁺⁺ |
|---|---|---|---|---|
| None | 409 | 19.5% | 7% | yes |
| Occasional | 375 | 17.8% | 70% | yes |
| Moderate | 134 | 6.4% | 11% | yes |
| Problem | 148 | 7.0% | 6% | no |
| Harmful | 1,035 | 49.3% | 6%** | yes |
| | 2,101*** | | | |

*Source*: *Goddard 1991: 26
⁺Table B (*ibid.*)
*Notes*: **according to Goddard (1991: 31) the percentage of harmful drinking is 11% in unskilled manual men (i.e. social class V) – this is also statistically significant; ⁺⁺chi squared at 0.05 significance level; ***HHELP data between early 1987 and June 1991.

step is assessing the motivation of the client. This is often better done by a counsellor, who will usually have more time, and sometimes more experience, than a general practitioner.

Easy access to alcohol detoxification facilities for those drinkers with alcohol dependency syndrome is essential (Edwards 1987). However, only a minority of problem drinkers seen by HHELP had such severe alcohol withdrawal symptoms that they needed detoxification. The majority of these who were detoxified returned to drinking.

There is a lot of evidence that those people with good social back-up, i.e. caring family, job and stable housing, do better than those without, in the long term. The street drinker is thus probably the most difficult patient with an alcohol problem to help. Despite this, most achieved some improvement in their health status while they were dry. Viewing successful therapy in terms of any improvement in the physical or mental state of the patient, however temporary, rather than a 'cure' may help the primary health care worker cope more positively with the patient's relapse!

Most of the clients encountered by HHELP are binge drinkers (estimated at least three-quarters). They tend to drink very heavily when they have money, usually just after they have received their benefit cheque. The rest of the time they drink intermittently. This pattern of drinking may explain some of the differences in morbidity between housed and homeless alcoholics. End-stage alcoholic cirrhosis is much rarer among homeless drinkers. Pollak (1975) suggested this may be because a binge drinker's liver has time to recover between binges.

Problems such as alcohol-related peripheral neuropathy (damaged nerves) and myopathy (damaged muscles) also occur. A co-factor in these problems must be poor nutrition. The complications of acute alcohol withdrawal, such as withdrawal epileptic fits and delirium tremens, also occur. There is also a well-recognized association between drinking and trauma (see Table 3.15, p. 84).

Minor degrees of brain damage related to alcohol are fairly common. The underlying causes for this are multifactorial. Repeated head injury, poor nutrition including vitamin deficiency (mainly the vitamin B group), the direct toxic effects of alcohol on brain cells and damage during epileptic fits all have a part to play. A psychologist attached to the HHELP team carried out cognitive tests on a number of homeless clients with alcohol problems. Short-term memory impairment was found to be the commonest problem. This may well militate against an individual's ability to cope with everyday tasks such as budgeting and remembering to pay rent. A larger study of the cognitive function of homeless people with drink problems needs to be carried out to elucidate the depth of these problems. Brain damage may also cause epilepsy. One completely unexpected benefit from cognitive testing was the agreement of a couple of local authorities to accept brain-damaged alcoholics as vulnerable.

HHELP did come across several individuals with more severe alcoholic brain damage, including alcoholic dementia (e.g. Korsakoff's Syndrome); sadly, numbered among these were a few patients aged 30 and under. Some of these had actually stopped drinking because of their brain damage – they had forgotten to drink! The scope for physical therapy is very limited, as this sort of damage is irreversible. The main problem for these people is a complete lack of appropriate shelter. HHELP encountered a number of local councils which do not accept alcoholics as vulnerable under the Housing Act even when they are severely disabled with alcoholic brain damage. When a council does agree to shelter them, this shelter is usually wholly inappropriate – bed and breakfast accommodation. Many of these people actually need some sort of specialist continuing care, in an environment where drinking may be tolerated. There is a great need for this sort of special supportive shelter in the United Kingdom.

The physical effect of alcohol can damage every organ in the body. Therapy needs to concentrate on the drinking problem and the physical symptoms. Many of HHELP's patients are poorly motivated to change their drinking patterns; despite this, they continue to need treatment for physical symptoms. Chest problems are more frequent among drinkers (Pollak 1975). Gastritis is also commoner. Antacids and drugs which block stomach acid secretion have an important role to play. The essential elements of good care for these patients are to be nonjudgemental, to take symptoms seriously and to treat the treatable. This approach can be very difficult if the patient is drunk! In 1990 just over 5 per cent of all clients consulting with the HHELP general practitioners were drunk. A pragmatic approach to this situation is to make sure there is no serious physical problem. However, assessing a patient's mental state when they are drunk remains problematic.

**Drugs**

The regular use of hard drugs in HHELP's patients is small, but it is increasing (see Table 3.13). In the East End of London the problem is mainly one of minor tranquillizers (benzodiazepines and chlormethiazole – 'Heminevrin') abuse.

Up to 10 per cent of all HHELP's patients have a problem with minor tranquillizers. The majority of this group also have an alcohol problem. Unfortunately, the supply of these drugs onto the streets comes mainly from the misuse of drugs prescribed by general practitioners. Why do GPs do it? Some feel that they genuinely do help a few patients with alcohol problems to detoxify. Others probably do it to 'please' the patient, as they can rarely solve their housing problem. This undoubtedly causes frustration on the part of some general practitioners and tranquillizers may seem to offer an easy option in a busy surgery setting. In addition, the patient may also put pressure on the doctor to prescribe. An attempt to ameliorate depression, anxiety or alcohol abuse then rapidly becomes a source of yet more problems.

As with alcohol abuse, most of the patients who abuse drugs do so in an intermittent fashion. Thus problems with withdrawal are not as severe as for someone who has a long-standing dependency. There are, however, a significant minority of patients who are dependent on minor tranquillizers. Therapy for these individuals is extremely difficult. Most have a mixed tranquillizer/alcohol problem. In East London the local alcohol detoxification unit does not routinely detoxify an alcoholic with a mixed dependency. A tranquillizer detoxification can take several weeks as compared with a week for most alcohol detoxifications. This would have resource implications if tranquillizer detoxifications were available on the National Health Service. The HHELP team has found that it is almost impossible to get such a detoxification, and on the whole the idea of a 'home' or a 'street' detoxification is untenable. One needs some form of stable

*Table 3.13* Types of drugs abused by 410 HHELP clients – four years till October 1991 (total population 3,015 individuals)*

| Type of drug** | No. of individuals | Percentage of total |
|---|---|---|
| benzodiazepines | 218 | 7.2 |
| cannabis | 184 | 6.1 |
| amphetamines*** | 172 | 5.7 |
| chlormethiazole* | 95 | 3.2 |
| cocaine | 65 | 2.2 |
| barbiturates | 55 | 1.8 |
| solvents | 43 | 1.4 |
| opiates | 43 | 1.4 |
| LSD | 3 | 0.1 |

*Notes*: *many individuals abused more than one drug; this table probably under-estimates the size of the drug problem;
**this table refers to regular drug abuse;
***most oral not intravenous use; the number of amphetamine abusers has increased dramatically recently;
˙also known as 'Heminevrin' – usually abused with benzodiazepines.

supportive environment for this to be effective. The Drug Dependency Units (DDU) in the National Health Service tend to be interested in 'hard' drugs (heroin, amphetamines and cocaine – usually intravenous use). In East London the local DDUs effectively offered no useful support to clients with mixed chemical dependency.

The commonest serious problems encountered by HHELP among mixed abusers were the consequences of overdoses of tranquillizers combined with alcohol. Sometimes the drugs were taken in their 'normal' therapeutic doses, but mixed with alcohol. More often they were taken in excess dose again mixed with alcohol. These overdoses were not usually a consequence of genuine suicidal intent. Every year there was a constant stream of deaths (see Table 3.15, p. 84) and attendances at hospital accident and emergency departments (at least one per month) from such overdoses. It is largely because of the consequences of these overdoses that the author does not believe it is safe to prescribe tranquillizers to unsupervised homeless patients who have a drink problem. The advent of pharmacy advisers to Family Health Services Authorities will prompt much closer scrutiny of the prescribing of tranquillizers especially to at risk groups such as the homeless.

Over the last two years there has been a doubling in the proportion of homeless people using amphetamines. The causes for this need further investigation. The amphetamine abusers are on the whole young and tend not to inject. Those homeless patients in East London who used hard drugs had all the medical conditions known to afflict drug users. For intravenous drug users these included skin infections, abscesses, thrombophlebitis and hepatitis. The incidence of HIV infection among HHELP's population of drug users is unknown.

**Teeth**

The dental problems of homeless people have until recently been neglected. However, the following discussion is based on the unpublished work of Blanaid Daly, a dentist at King's College Dental School. Dental care is a very low priority for the homeless as access to general dentists is restricted for many of the same reasons as access to general practitioners. Many homeless people are able to get treatment when they have a dental emergency either from local dental practitioners or from a dental hospital. Non-emergency work seems to be more difficult to obtain.

Hopes (1985) found that single homeless men and women had a low level of perceived need despite having increased dental disease. This may in part explain the relatively low demand for, and use of, dental services. Many homeless people expect to have unsightly dentition and to lose their teeth.

Most homeless people are entitled to free dental treatment under the National Health Service; however, many homeless people are not aware of their rights. If a client is not claiming income support they have to fill in a form before they can receive free treatment. There is then a three-week wait before the treatment is sanctioned. Often clients will need help filling in this form. A survey of homeless people in East London (unpublished – HHELP/NFA) showed an almost 50 per cent illiteracy rate – in itself a barrier to care.

Another barrier to accessing dental personnel may be unfavourable attitudes by these workers (Burgess – dental student project, unpublished). Most dentists run appointment systems and homeless people often find these difficult to use. Some dentists do not invite homeless people back for follow-up care, under circumstances where housed patients would be. This may indicate that different standards are being applied to homeless people. Another indicator of this is the excess number of pulled teeth which results from dental work with the homeless. This involves a single contact with the patient, thus avoiding the need for further appointments.

*Table 3.14* Main types of dental problems found among homeless clients
(breakdown by age)

| Age range (years) | Problems | Possible causes |
|---|---|---|
| <30 | lots of tartar<br>wisdom teeth impaction<br>– often with infections<br>removal of teeth necessary<br>rampant caries<br>dental phobia | poor dental care<br>inferior tooth<br>  brushes or none<br>malnutrition |
| 30–50 | lots of tartar<br>unusual pattern of caries<br>– lots of pitting<br>lots of chronic irritation<br>– broken teeth<br>– plenty of calculus<br>– many holes | poor dental care<br>smoking<br>alcohol<br>malnutrition<br>infrequent visits<br>  to dentists |
| >50 | poor dentures*<br>a few rotten teeth left*<br>other oral pathology | all the above<br>difficulty getting<br>  dentures made˙ |

*Source*: Blanaid Daly
*Notes*: *leads to difficulty eating properly;
˙ dentists may not be paid for making dentures.

The published information about the dental health of homeless
people in Britain is very limited and describes the problems of hostel
dwellers. This work shows that the older homeless attend dentists very
infrequently. Daly's work with younger homeless people suggests that
they are much more likely to visit a dentist than older ones. Those on
the streets were less likely to be treated. Again, this follows the pattern
of access to general medical practitioners.

In Table 3.14 there is a summary of the dental problems of homeless
people by age. This work was carried out at Crisis at Christmas and a
number of South London day centres for the homeless by Blanaid
Daly.

Many of the treatments needed for these problems are fairly simple;
for example, most younger patients just need descaling and polishing.
Explaining the importance of dental care to the single homeless is
important. This may involve some outreach work. Advocacy is also
important, for example, helping patients make appointments with
ordinary dental practitioners.

## Nutrition

Many homeless people depend on charitable hand-outs from day centres and hostels for some or all of their meals. The quality and variety of the food they eat is thus in the hands of others. Homeless people have little 'consumer' choice. Food is often donated by the supermarket chains and is usually near or past its expiry date. It is often then stored in inadequate refrigerators. The risks attached to such practices are obvious. It is not surprising therefore that there is a higher incidence of food poisoning among HHELP's homeless patients.

The meals offered in many hostels and day centres are also nutritionally unbalanced. This is an area where the influence of a dietician and other primary health care workers can be very useful. For example, following a report by a dietician on the food offered by St Botolph's Crypt, East London, to its homeless clients in the evenings, several changes were instituted. These included ensuring brown bread and salad sandwiches were always available. Some of the local East End hostels have also been encouraged to offer less fried food and more salads and vegetable dishes at meal times. Unfortunately this latter initiative has had variable success. Vitamin deficiency can occur. Drinkers are at greater risk of this, partly because of poor diet but also because of poorer gut absorption due to alcoholic damage.

Poor nutrition places patients at greater risk of infections, in particular of the respiratory tract. The increased incidence of dental problems is also partly a reflection of poor nutrition. A more detailed study of the nutritional problems of the single homeless in Britain needs to be undertaken to clarify exactly what sorts of measures are needed to improve nutritional status.

## Feet

Only a small proportion of HHELP consultations (4 per cent of the author's in 1989) involved foot problems as the presenting complaint. The reason for this low figure is the regular services of Maureen Docherty, an outreach chiropodist in one of the centres. A detailed audit of her work was undertaken in 1982 (Toon *et al.* 1987). During this period she saw over a hundred individuals and found,

> many of the patients' chiropody problems were due to poor footwear which was often ill-fitting, worn and not waterproof. Plastic shoes with no ventilation and cheap nylon socks, together

with constant walking and hyperhidrosis led to gross maceration and blistering, the most common severe problem. Ulcers resulted from a variety of causes – pressure from thick nails, break downs underlying hard corns, neglected burns or injuries to the feet . . . sixteen cases of foot deformity were seen.

Docherty found that most (58 per cent) of the patients seen had had good foot hygiene; however, almost a quarter had more severe problems. These figures need to be viewed carefully as the clients were mainly self-referrals and, as such, were not a representative sample of the users of St Botolph's Crypt evening centre.

Easy access to chiropody services is important for the homeless. Sometimes this involves some outreach work. Usually, however, a friendly chiropodist working in a normal setting who is flexible about seeing people without appointments is all that is needed. Most district chiropody services offer some sort of domiciliary service. Homeless people should be included in this.

## Trauma

The incidence of trauma among homeless people is much the same as that in the average population (see Table 3.7, p. 62). However, homeless people do tend to have more severe trauma and also probably under-report minor trauma. The commonest problems found in East London were bruises, sprains, superficial burns, lacerations and contusions. These types of problems are due to a combination of a number of factors, violent crime, poor basic living conditions, alcohol and drug abuse being the most prevalent. Sadly, the incidence of violent death is also fairly high. Table 3.15 illustrates the deaths among HHELP patients in 1988 (Whaley *et al.* 1989: Appendix 1: 20). This must be an underestimate, because HHELP was not informed about all the deaths.

## Chronic disease

This is an area where there are significant differences from the housed population. The conditions not covered elsewhere include cardiovascular disease, rheumatological disorders, physical disability, cancer and diabetes. All these, with the exception of rheumatological problems, were less frequent than would have been expected (Table 3.7, p. 62). This ties in with the analysis of Shanks (1988). It is not clear why chronic disease should be less prevalent in the single

*Table 3.15* Deaths of HHELP patients in 1988

| Number | Cause |
|--------|-------|
| 4 | burns[+] |
| 3 | heart attack (one[+]) |
| 3 | inhalation of vomit with alcohol & drug overdose*[+] |
| 2 | subdural haematoma (brain haemorrhage after a blow to the head)[+] |
| 2 | cancer |
| 2 | unknown |
| 1 | hypothermia |
| 1 | murdered |
| 1 | pulmonary TB (complicated by hypothermia)[+] |
| 1 | malnutrition & hypothermia[+] |
| 1 | candidal endocarditis (related malnutrition not to HIV infection) |
| 1 | drowning & drug overdose*[+] |

*Source*: Whaley *et al.* 1989: Appendix 1: 20
*Notes*: *all these overdoses were with minor tranquillizers;
[+]these patients were known to drink heavily.

homeless population. Perhaps one factor is that most local authorities would accept people suffering with these diseases as being vulnerable and in priority need. They may therefore never reach the stage of being homeless. Another reason may be that some of these problems are undiagnosed (Featherstone and Ashmore 1988: 354). More research needs to be done into the reasons for different disease patterns in sub-populations of the homeless.

In the future the prevalence of HIV infection will rise. Given current interpretations of the Housing Act it seems doubtful whether a person with AIDS or AIDS-related complex would be refused shelter by a local authority. However, asymptomatic carriers of the virus may not be deemed as in priority need by some local authorities even though it is now recognized that high levels of stress and heavy alcohol consumption (Siegel 1991) can lead to a more rapid progression of the disease.

## Health promotion and prevention

These are both high on the government's agenda for primary care. The introduction of the new general practitioner contract (*Working for Patients* 1989) with its targets for smears and immunizations and extra payments for health promotion clinics illustrates this. For most homeless people health promotion and prevention is a very low priority. Until recently the medical services aimed at the single homeless have been reactive. Things are beginning to change. In Figure 3.5 (see p. 65), there is a breakdown of the outcome of all consultations with the HHELP general practitioners in 1990. Just over 13 per cent of all consultation outcomes included health promotion or prevention activities. This is still too low but at least it is a start.

The rest of this section will identify a few areas where health promotional activities may benefit homeless patients.

*Health surveillance*

There is considerable evidence that homeless people have more untreated disease than the housed population (e.g. Featherstone and Ashmore 1988). Opportunistic screening for conditions such as chronic bronchitis, dental caries, poor hearing especially in the older patients, indigestion, poor visual acuity, feet and skin problems are likely to reveal pathology amenable to therapy. This is likely to improve the quality of life for these individuals. To carry out these sorts of activities the staff in the hostels or day centres must be committed and enthusiastic so as to encourage their clients to attend for surveillance, particularly as screening is time consuming. The health worker involved in screening, often a nurse specialist, will be aware that some patients could be identified as severely disabled and thus qualify as vulnerable under the Housing Act. This might be the first step on the road to more secure accommodation.

*Immunization*

It is important to ensure that homeless people are up to date with their immunizations, in particular tetanus. Homeless people are more vulnerable to the effects of influenza and therefore annual flu vaccination campaigns should be undertaken in centres used by homeless people.

*Advice*

It is the role of the primary health care worker to discuss issues such as smoking, drinking, nutrition, keeping warm and personal safety with their patients. It is well recognized that such advice and counselling can lead to a change in behaviour. This must apply to homeless

*Table 3.16* Risk factors for abnormal cervical smears

| Risk factor | No. | Percentage |
|---|---|---|
| Smokers | 42 | 84 |
| More than ten sexual partners* | 19 | 38 |
| Onset sexual activity less than sixteen years of age⁺ | 12 | 26 |
| Never used barrier contraception | 22 | 44 |
| History of wart virus infection | 3 | 6 |

*Notes*: *three women had had more than 500 partners;
⁺seven women had been sexually abused as children.

patients as well. The efficacy of such advice needs to be studied further in relationship to the homeless.

*Cervical cytology*

Two members of the HHELP team (Balazs and Whaley) with the help of Dr Fran Reader (previous appointment Consultant in Family Planning Tower Hamlets Health Authority) carried out a survey of the cervical smear status of fifty consecutive women consulting with the team in 1989. A detailed look at the findings illustrate many of the problems of caring for homeless women. Women who were homeless, aged between 20 and 65 years, excluding those with a hysterectomy, were recruited. Each woman was asked about risk factors for abnormal cervical smears (Table 3.16).

In Figure 3.6 there is a breakdown of previous smear history. The results of this audit are worrying. One-third of the women who had had smears did not know the results. Of those who did know their smear results two had very abnormal smears (CIN III). One of these women had been lost to follow-up, the other had been adequately treated. Twenty women were offered smears: twelve of these had never had a smear before, seven had had a smear but more than five years previously and one had had a swab taken previously, not a smear as she thought. The total number of smears taken was seven. The results of these smears were another CIN III and one vaginal tract infection (trichomonas vaginalis). Thirteen women who were offered smears refused (Table 3.17). Nine of these women had never had a smear.

The conclusions of this small study were that homeless women are possibly more at risk of having abnormal smears, but that they are less likely to have had smears and, even if they did, they often did not know the result. This study is therefore a good illustration of the

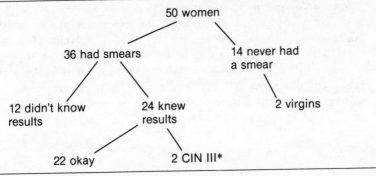

*Note:* *highly abnormal smear result – needing urgent treatment.

*Figure 3.6* Previous smear history

*Table 3.17* Women who refused to have smears

| Reason | Number |
|---|---|
| No female smear taker available | 4 |
| Menstruating | 1 |
| Afraid | 1 |
| Acute psychosis* | 1 |
| Lesbian | 1 |
| Korsakoff's Syndrome* | 1 |
| Too embarrassed | 1 |
| No reason (mute)* | 1 |
| Vaginismus | 1 |
| Too unwell˙ | 1 |
| Total | 13 |

*Notes:* *unable to gain informed consent;
˙ dying of end-stage alcoholic cirrhosis.

'inverse care law' (Tudor Hart 1971). To overcome these deficiencies the following procedures were instituted for all smears taken by HHELP:

– each smear delivered to the laboratory on the same day
– smears specially labelled and processed within five working days
– results back to HHELP within two weeks
– FHSA computerized recall system cancelled (it was unable to cope with NFA as an address!) and a separate manual system set up
– all previous results confirmed by phone or writing
– each patient asked how they wanted to be contacted with their result
– rapid colposcopy appointments

women accompanied to colposcopy.

Since these changes were instituted, the one major problem with taking cervical smears has been the refusal of some women to have them. This has been slightly eased by the presence of more women doctors on the team. The above system involves a lot of work which may mean that some GPs could be disinclined to register homeless women, particularly if their practices are near their cervical cytology targets.

### Safer sex

One of the results of this work with cervical cytology was the realization that our patients were at risk of sexually transmitted diseases and some women at risk of unwanted pregnancy. Most younger patients are now counselled about safer sexual practices. Condoms have been made available at some of the centres. To prevent the spread of HIV and hepatitis B infection the message of safer sex must be taken to the homeless, particularly the young.

### Contraception

This must be discussed with homeless clients in the same way as for housed ones.

## CONCLUSIONS

Alan, a 25-year-old, who was homeless for eight years before being resettled, considers a 'home' as being where 'I've got the key to the door so I've got independence. I've also got the option whether I want to cook or eat out. I've got my bed there so I don't have to worry about where I'm going to sleep so it's secure. I'm secure. No one can throw me out.'

Ideally, access to secure affordable accommodation should be a therapeutic outcome for all homeless people, one in which the intervention of primary health care workers can be an important enabling influence. While the single homeless have many medical problems, most are compounded by homelessness. This population also have specific health problems which have been detailed in this chapter. On the whole these are best treated by multidisciplinary teams with access to wider paramedical and counselling support. Because single homeless men and women encounter difficulties in gaining access to services these teams sometimes need to adopt an outreach approach to reach those most at risk. The optimal treatment of some conditions also requires admission to beds where good quality nursing care is available, preferably outside the setting of a large hospital.

More research is needed into the patterns of morbidity among the single homeless. The special problems of homeless women also need to be explored. Work needs to be carried out to study which sorts of therapeutic interventions are most effective. In consequence, those working with the homeless need to be constantly auditing their work. One way to overcome the lack of clinical information about homeless people would be to give them their own records. This should be tried on a large scale.

The health care needs of homeless people are constantly changing. This is partly a reflection of demographic changes (e.g. more young women), changes of central government policy (e.g. increased emphasis on health promotion) and changes in disease patterns. The deliverers of health care must be aware of these factors and adjust their clinical practices when necessary. For example, it is now apparent that the best way to screen for tuberculosis is by clinical case finding not by mass X-ray screening.

Health prevention and promotion are areas where the single homeless have in the past been neglected. Cervical cytology illustrates some of the difficulties of delivering this service to homeless women. To provide a level of care equivalent to that for housed women considerably more time and effort needs to be expended by their carers. Although prevention is a low priority for homeless people, it must be a high priority for their carers.

Health care workers would benefit from extra training in specific problems of homelessness. An important role for carers is advocacy. This is one of the ways of breaking down the barriers to access to mainstream services. In the East End of London the main cause of non-registration of homeless people with general practitioners is not the refusal of GPs to take them onto their lists but their failure to attempt to register. This failure to use general practitioners is a strong argument in favour of a flexible outreach primary health care service.

## ACKNOWLEDGEMENTS

I should like to thank all members of the HHELP team, the users and staff of the voluntary sector in East London, Alan Bennett – general manager of the City & East London Family Health Services Authority, the Department of Health and Jenny Law.

# REFERENCES

Bull, G. M. and Morton, J. (1978) 'Relationships of temperature and death rates from all causes and from certain respiratory and arteriosclerotic diseases in different age groups', *Age and Aging* 7: 210.

Burgess, D. (1986) 'The dental health needs of homeless men: what are they and how can they be met?', unpublished paper, King's College Hospital School of Dentistry.

*Code of Guidance* (revised 1983) accompanying the 1977 Housing (Homeless Persons) Act.

Committee on Health Care for Homeless People (1988) *Homelessness, Health, and Human Needs*, Institute of Medicine, Washington, DC: National Academic Press, pp. 45–7.

Connelly, J. *et al.* (1991) *Housing or Homelessness: A Public Health Perspective*, London: Royal Colleges of Physicians of the United Kingdom.

Curwen, M. and Davis, T. (1988) 'Winter mortality, temperature and influenza: has the relationship changed in recent years?', *Population Trends* 54: 17–20.

Edwards, G. (1987) *Treatment of Drinking Problems: A Guide for the Helping Professions*, second edition, Oxford: Blackwell Scientific Publications, pp. 330–5.

Featherstone P. and Ashmore, C. (1988) 'Health surveillance project among single homeless men in Bristol', *Journal of the Royal College of General Practitioners* 88: 353–5.

Goddard, E. (1991) *Drinking in England and Wales in the Late 1980s*, London: Social Survey Division of OPCS; pp. 24–32.

Hopes, I. (1985) *The Dental Health Needs for Dental Care of Homeless and Rootless People Living in Three London Boroughs with Reference to their Social and Medical Backgrounds*, London: Camberwell Health Authority.

*Housing Vulnerable Young Single People* (1989) National Children's Home Research Report, London: National Children's Home.

Lowry, S. (1991) *Housing and Health*, London: British Medical Journal.

Martin, C.J. and Platt, S.D. (1987) 'Housing conditions and Ill-health', *British Medical Journal* 294: 1125.

Mitchell, R.E. (1976) 'Cultural and health influences on building, housing and community, standards: cost implications for the human habitat', *Human Ecology* 4: 297–330.

*Morbidity Statistics from General Practice, Second National Study 1970–71* (1982), London: HMSO (Royal College of General Practitioners, OPCS & DHSS).

*Morbidity Statistics from General Practice, Third National Study 1981–2* (1986), London: HMSO (Royal College of General Practitioners, OPCS & DHSS).

NFA (1986) *Action for a Change*, London: No Fixed Abode.

*A Nice Way to Treat People* (1987) British Broadcasting Corporation, p. 2.

Pollak, B. (1975) *Proceedings of the Royal Society of Medicine* 68: 13.

Powell, P.V. (1988) 'Editorial: Primary health care for the single homeless', *British Medical Journal* 297: 84–5.

Ramsden, S.S. *et al.* (1988) 'Tuberculosis among the central London homeless', *Journal of the Royal College of General Practitioners* 22(1): 16–17.

Randall, G. (1989) *Homeless and Hungry: A Sign of the Times*, London: Centrepoint Soho, Central Office.

Rapley, M., Balazs, J. and Burd, M. (1991) 'Down and out in the East End of London: defining a role for the clinical psychologist working with single homeless people. Part I – The homeless man: a psychological enigma?', *Clinical Psychology Forum* February: 2–5.

Reuler, J. B. and Balazs, J. R. (1991) 'Portable medical record for the homeless mentally ill', *British Medical Journal* 303: 446.

Richards, J. (ed.) (1989) *Tower Hamlets People*, Department of Community Medicine, Tower Hamlets Health Authority, p. 11.

Roth L.H. *et al.* (1986) 'Homelessness and mental health policy; developing an appropriate role for the 1980s', *Community Mental Health Journal* 22(3): 303–14.

Schmidt, W. and de Lint, J.Q. (1969) 'Mortality experiences of male and female alcoholics', *Quarterly Journal of Studies in Alcohol* 30: 112.

Secretaries of State for Health (1989) *Working for Patients*, Command 555, London: HMSO.

Shanks, N.J. (1988) 'Medical morbidity of the homeless', *Journal of Epidemiology and Community Health* 42: 183–6.

Shever, M.A., Black, M., Victor, C., Benzeval, M., Gill, M. and Judge, K. (1991) *Homelessness and Utilization of Acute Hospital Services in London*, London: Kings Fund.

Siegel, L. (1991) 'Alcohol and AIDS: a clinical perspective', *Alcoholism* 3: 1–2.

Single Homeless in London (1990) *Primary Health Care for Homeless People in London: A Strategic Approach*, report of the health sub-group of the joint working party on single homeless in London, London: London Borough of Hammersmith and Fulham, p. 21.

Skinner, C. *et al.* (1990) 'Control and prevention of tuberculosis in Britain: an updated code of practice', sub-committee of the Joint Tuberculosis Committee of the British Thoracic Society, *British Medical Journal* 300: 995–9.

Smellie, J. *et al.* (1991) *HHELP 1990 Annual Report and Review of 1987–89*, London: East London Homeless Health Team.

*Social Trends 21* (1991) London: HMSO, p. 121.

Stern, R., Stilwell, B. and Heuston, J. (1988) *From the Margins to the Mainstream: Collaboration in Planning Services with Single Homeless People*, London: West Lambeth Health Authority, Priority Services Unit, Appendix K.

Stevens, S. *et al.* (1991) 'The public health management of tuberculosis among the single homeless – is mass miniature X-ray screening effective?', *Journal of Epidemiology and Community Health* 46: 141–3.

Timms, P.W. (1989) 'Homelessness and mental illness', *Health Trends* 21: 70–1.

Toon, P.D., Thomas, K. and Doherty, M. (1987) 'Audit of work at a medical centre for the homeless over one year', *Journal of the Royal College of General Practitioners* 37: 120–2.

'Tuberculosis and the alcoholic' (1978) *Lancet* 26 August: 460–1.

Tudor Hart, J. (1971) 'The inverse care law', *Lancet* 1.

Weller, B. *et al.* (1987) 'Crisis at Christmas', *Lancet* 2: 553.

Whaley, K. *et al.* (1989) *The Future of Primary Health Care for the Single Homeless in East London*, London: City & East London Family Practitioner Committee and No Fixed Abode.

*Wytham Hall Annual Report 1989–90* (1990) London: Wytham Hall.

## APPENDIX A: THE GROUPING OF ACCOMMODATION STATUS USED IN THIS CHAPTER

| | *Accommodation types* | |
|---|---|---|
| 1. | No Fixed Abode | – rough/sleeping on the streets |
| 2. | Unstable including: temporary | – squat<br>night-shelter<br>resettlement unit<br>short-stay hostel<br>with friends/relatives<br>hotel/bed & breakfast |
| | Long-stay hostel | – (most of the published literature includes all hostel dwellers as living in temporary accommodation) |
| 3. | Stable (secure) | – private rented<br>council<br>housing association<br>owner-occupier |
| 4. | Other | – prison<br>specialist – alcohol<br>       – drug<br>       – psychiatric |

## APPENDIX B: ALCOHOL – UNITS PER WEEK AND DEGREES OF HARM

| | Units per week | |
|---|---|---|
| | *Women* | *Men* |
| None | 0 | 0 |
| Occasional/light | 1 <14 | 1<21 |
| Moderate | 15<25 | 22<35 |
| Problem/fairly heavy | 26<35 | 36<50 |
| Harmful/very heavy | >36 | >51 |

*Source*: Goddard 1991: 27

# APPENDIX C: CONTROL OF TUBERCULOSIS AMONG STAFF WORKING WITH THE SINGLE HOMELESS IN EAST LONDON

1. All new staff and volunteers coming into regular contact with the homeless should have a pre-employment medical. This should include a questionnaire. If suspicious symptoms are picked up, the person should have a chest X-ray before starting work. Everyone else should have a Heaf test (looking for immunity to tuberculosis). Those with negative tests should have BCGs before starting work. Staff must be warned that the BCG will not provide protection for six to eight weeks. Those with very strong reactions should have chest X-rays. If the chest X-ray is normal no further action is required unless the person is a member of a high risk ethnic group, or there are clinical grounds to suspect recent infection.

2. Examination of contacts is a useful exercise. Close contacts, especially when the patient has the tuberculous bacillus in their sputum need close follow-up. The examination includes an inquiry into BCG vaccination status, Heaf testing and chest X-ray. Patients with very weak (grade 0) Heaf tests under the age of 35 should be offered BCG vaccination following a second Heaf test. Antituberculous chemoprophylaxis may be considered in those with a strongly positive Heaf test. Examination of close contacts is probably best done by a local chest clinic. Most occupational contacts (such as hostel workers) are much less likely to develop tuberculosis. These less intimate or casual contacts make up the vast majority of staff working with the homeless. They probably do not need such rigorous screening. All the staff need to do is to follow the advice in paragraph 3 (below).

3. Staff who develop chest symptoms should attend their general practitioners. The threshold for carrying out chest X-rays should be low, as should be the threshold for referring to a chest physician. There is no clinical rationale for yearly chest X-rays of all staff in the absence of a clinical indication. Routine period chest X-rays are unnecessary but an X-ray should be taken if an employee develops suspicious symptoms (for example, an unexplained cough lasting more than three weeks, persistent fever or weight loss).

4. All staff should have a chest X-ray on leaving regular work with the homeless. This has more to do with employer liability than good clinical care.

# 4 Mental health and homelessness

*Philip Timms*

## INTRODUCTION

The recent wave of interest in and concern about the plight of homeless people with mental health problems has originated from two sources.

Over the last five years in Britain a wider awareness of homelessness issues has arisen among both professionals and lay people, not as a product of academic studies or the sterling efforts of the numerous voluntary organizations involved, but simply generated by the increasing numbers of visibly homeless people on the streets of our cities and major towns. Of these, a substantial number appear, even to the general public, to be psychologically distressed or disturbed.

In parallel with the higher profile of homelessness issues, there has been increasing concern about the fate of patients discharged from psychiatric hospitals into the 'community' as part of the programme of hospital closures. Psychiatrists are said to be discharging patients out of the old institutions without adequate or appropriate community support. They are then left to fend for themselves, may relapse and for many reasons lose their accommodation and become homeless.

These two distinct social processes have become linked in the public mind, producing a simple explanatory model – long-stay patients are being decanted from the hospitals into an ill-prepared community and, from there, briskly on to the streets.

However, this explanation makes several assumptions – that the phenomenon of the homeless mentally ill is new, that psychiatric bed closures have happened only recently and that discharges from long-stay beds are typically unplanned. I hope to demonstrate that these assumptions are false. The real situation is more messy, less related to closure of psychiatric beds and more to do with the way in which psychiatry is practised in the post-institutional era.

## HISTORY

One of the first, albeit oblique, mentions of the homeless mentally ill is to be found in an Act of Parliament concerned with the management of vagrancy in general, the Vagrancy Act of 1714 (29) (Allderidge 1979). This empowered Justices of the Peace to confine 'Persons of little or no Estates, who, by Lunacy, or otherwise, are furiously mad, and dangerous to be permitted to go abroad'. It also empowered them to return to their parish of origin anyone so confined who did not belong to the parish or town in which they were arrested.

From then until the Second World War very little seems to have been written on the subject in this country. Even George Orwell (1933) does not seem to have noticed any madness in his perambulations through the world of the destitute in the London and Paris of the 1930s, although he does seem to have noticed those he termed 'simple-minded' who today would almost certainly be regarded as having learning difficulties. However, psychiatrists have periodically interested themselves in the relationship between homelessness and mental illness for nearly a century.

The first to address the issue directly was a German psychiatrist, Wilmanns, in 1906. At this time in Germany, vagrancy was an offence and those who could not demonstrate that they had a home to go to could be arrested and confined in the police workhouse. He noticed that many of the homeless so detained were transferred to his hospital from the local workhouse. In his survey of these patients he found 120 homeless men and women who had been committed with a diagnosis of schizophrenia. There was no more work done on the specific relationship between homelessness and mental illness for many years. However, interest in the relationship between social conditions and psychiatric illnesses had begun to grow, particularly in the USA. Faris and Dunham (1939) suggested that the prevalence of mental illness was higher in what they called 'the disorganised community'.

Two psychiatrists, one American and one French, even produced roughly equivalent descriptive classifications of the homeless:

|  | *Anderson (1923)* | *Vexliard (1957)* |
|---|---|---|
| Itinerant workers: | Hobos | Errants |
| Itinerant non-workers | Tramps | Vagabonds |
| Non-itinerant non-workers: | Bums | Clochards |

Neither of these served either science or the homeless to any degree. More significantly and helpfully, Bogue, a sociologist, looked at the inhabitants of Chicago's Skid Row in 1956 (Bogue 1963). Although alcoholism was his main focus (and indeed he found a very high rate of alcoholism) he also noted that roughly 1 in 5 of the men he interviewed was suffering from 'mental illness' or 'mental and nervous trouble' of some description.

Post-war interest in this country was aroused by Stuart Whiteley's review of a series of acute male admissions to a South London observation ward (Whiteley 1955). He noted that 8 per cent were of no fixed abode, a much higher proportion than would be expected from the numbers of homeless men in the local area. He diagnosed around a third as suffering from schizophrenia, mostly with delusional ideas. He noted that, compared with homeless men with other diagnoses, those suffering from schizophrenia tended to be living in the most impoverished circumstances, such as night-shelters, rather than common lodging houses. His view was that, for his patients, 'the main cause [of homelessness] is the personality defect which does not allow him to form relationships'. He went on to recommend that:

> When he falls ill, the down and out should, ideally, be treated in a separate institution . . . where his environment was as near his normal habitat as possible. He would then be more likely to stay . . . it would be an advantage if he could be committed to the institution for a definite period, and as so many appear in court, this should be possible.
>
> (Whiteley 1955)

A curious mixture of the zoological and the coercive.

By the time Birmingham psychiatrists Berry and Orwin (1966) conducted a survey of admissions, 23 per cent of their acute male admissions were of no fixed abode. In addition, they noted that this proportion was rising fast compared with that in non-urban hospitals in their region. Seventy-four per cent of these homeless patients had previous hospital admissions. The authors commented:

> Their plight is evidence that the initial enthusiasm evoked by the new act (1959 Mental Health Act) for the discharge of psychotics into the community was premature and has resulted in the overwhelming of community services.
>
> Re-development of the centre of Birmingham has resulted in a reduction in the number of lodgings available for persons of no fixed abode.
>
> (Berry and Orwin 1966: 1026, 1027)

Their identification of the themes of inadequate community care and

*Table 4.1* British hostel surveys

| Survey | Schizophrenia | Alcoholism | Affective disorder | Personality disorder |
|---|---|---|---|---|
| Edwards *et al.* 1968 | 24 per cent | 25 per cent | N/K | N/K |
| Priest 1971 | 32 per cent | 18 per cent | 5 per cent | 18 per cent |
| Lodge Patch 1971 | 15 per cent | N/K | 8 per cent | 51 per cent |
| Tidmarsh and Wood 1972 | ~25 per cent | 25 per cent | ~5 per cent | 17 per cent |

lack of low-cost housing was prescient, but their recommendation of 'further investigation' bore little fruit.

Awareness among psychiatrists was growing, however. These first studies were both surveys of those who had managed to get into hospital. Griffith Edwards in London was the first to survey a hostel,[10] interviewing (with a team, it must be said) the entire population of the Camberwell Reception centre on one night (Edwards *et al.* 1968). He found that the proportion of those who had been admitted to mental hospital, 25 per cent, equalled the proportion of those with alcohol problems. This was perhaps the first hint that the traditional view of 'vagrancy' as characterized by alcoholism might be mistaken.

This evidence for a high prevalence of mental illness in the homeless population was confirmed by Ian Lodge Patch's 1970 doorstep survey of two Salvation Army hostels for men (Lodge Patch 1971). He diagnosed 15 per cent as suffering from schizophrenia and an astounding 50 per cent as being personality disordered. As his evaluations were based on one-off interviews, it seems highly likely that many of these men were actually suffering from schizophrenia. He again commented on community care: 'The small number of schizophrenics who were receiving treatment suggests both a failure of community care and inappropriately early discharge.' He also made some eminently sensible suggestions about co-ordinating homelessness hostels and night-shelters with the psychiatric services, but these were never taken up.

Robin Priest's 1971 Edinburgh survey approached the problem from a slightly different angle, comparing a general survey of the homeless population with those who were actually admitted to hospital. Compared with men with alcoholic problems or those with personality disorders, those with a diagnosis of schizophrenia (32 per cent of his population survey) tended not to find their way to treatment services.

In fact, over the last twenty years, successive surveys in British hostels (Tidmarsh and Wood 1972), night-shelters (Weller 1986) and prisons (Gunn 1974) have demonstrated the presence of large numbers of homeless men with schizophrenia. Moreover, there has been a significant absence of those less severe anxiety and depressive disorders which characterize the bulk of the psychiatric symptomatology presenting in a general practice setting.

There have been no equivalent studies of homeless women, although a survey of homeless women admitted to an East London psychiatric unit (Herzberg 1987) suggested a more profound level of disturbance than for those domiciled women admitted to the same unit.

Throughout these investigations, the numbers of men suffering from schizophrenia have been found at least to equal and sometimes to exceed the numbers of those with alcoholic problems. These figures suggest that the widely held view of homelessness as characterized by alcoholism is mistaken. Hospital admission rates have been noted to be excessive since the 1950s and it was suggested as long ago as 1966 that the over-representation of schizophrenia in this population was a consequence of inappropriate hospital discharge policy.

These findings are not unique to this country, but have been replicated on a larger scale in the USA (Bassuk 1984; Lamb 1984) where the Kennedy reforms of the mid-1960s produced a massive programme of deinstitutionalization with the expectation that community mental health centres would take the place of the old asylums in the care of the mentally ill. In Italy, 12 per cent of the patients deinstitutionalized under the 1978 legislation may now be homeless (Becker 1985).

So, the last thirty years of study of the homeless populations in the British Isles have suggested that the pre-eminent mental health problem in this setting is psychotic disorder, schizophrenia in particular. But is this still the case?

## RECENT WORK

In 1986–7 a survey was carried out at a Salvation Army hostel in South East London (Timms and Fry 1989). The impetus for this survey came from a local consultant psychiatrist, who had become aware of an increase in the number of homeless men being admitted to his ward. His impression was echoed by local Salvation Army staff. They were conscious of having to deal with large numbers of psychologically disturbed people, without having the necessary training or experience.

For practical reasons it was not possible to carry out a survey of the whole hostel. In addition, there was an idea around that the hostel was seeing a younger, more disturbed group of the mentally ill than had been the case previously. So, two groups were identified – those who had been there for more than a year and those who had newly arrived at the hostel. In the end, sixty-four new arrivals were interviewed and almost the whole 'resident' group of fifty-nine men. Both groups fitted into the picture of the 'traditional homeless' identified in previous surveys – white, working class, middle-aged, unemployed, with many men from Ireland and Scotland.

There was actually no significant difference between the two groups as far as age. Around 30 per cent of each group fulfilled the criteria for a diagnosis of schizophrenia – around ninety times the number expected from the rate in the general population. Of the men thus diagnosed, four-fifths were experiencing positive symptoms such as delusions, hallucinations and thought disorder. Curiously, there was very little 'minor' mental illness and little alcoholism – the latter because the local drinkers tended to gravitate to another local hostel which had a more liberal policy on drinking. Most of those with diagnosable disorders had had considerable contact with psychiatric services in the past, although most were not in contact with any psychiatric service at the time of interview.

Given this high prevalence of psychiatric disorder, there are issues about whether mental illness precedes and causes homelessness, or whether it is the stress of being homeless that precipitates psychiatric disorder. In all the cases in this survey the psychiatric disorder had preceded the loss of accommodation. The idea that newly arriving schizophrenics would be a younger, more disturbed group was not supported – there was no difference in ages and both groups had equal numbers and severity of symptoms.

One issue this survey did not address was the degree of handicap that those patients identified were experiencing. A survey conducted in Oxford (Marshall 1989) identified a large proportion of the residents as suffering from a level of handicap similar to that of long-stay patients in a local mental hospital.

Neither of these surveys addressed the problems of homeless women, traditionally a much less visible group. Nevertheless, it appears that the situation has not changed significantly over the last thirty years and that significant numbers of people with long-term mental health problems become homeless.

## ORIGINS OF HOMELESSNESS SPECIFIC TO THE MENTALLY ILL

### Hospital issues

*Hospital closures*

The recent spate of mental hospital bed closures has been cited as the main reason for the increasing numbers of homeless mentally ill people on the streets. The spectre has been raised of long-stay patients being turned out with nowhere and nobody to go to. However, the process of psychiatric deinstitutionalization has been going on for at least thirty years. The decline in the number of psychiatric beds in the Health Service started in 1954 when there were over 150,000 beds in asylums. There are now 77,628 beds devoted to psychiatry in England and Wales (*NHS Hospital Administrative Statistics*, 1990), some in old hospitals, many now in district general hospitals and teaching hospitals. Half of the bed losses were accomplished before 1970. Moreover, in both the Blackfriars survey carried out at a Salvation Army hostel mentioned above and in the US it has been noted that most of the homeless mentally ill have *not* been ex-long-stay patients, but have had repeated, relatively brief admissions (Appleby 1985). References to the inadequacy of community provision were being made as far back as 1966, and these may well explain the earlier hostel findings of a high prevalence of schizophrenia. They do not explain the recent apparent increases in the numbers of the homeless mentally ill on the street.

*Inadequate acute beds*

Figures for bed closures in acute units are hard to come by as the DoH statistics do not discriminate between mental hospitals and district hospitals or between acute and long-stay beds. However, it does seem that every Inner-London psychiatric service has had to close acute beds over the last five years. This means that, with bed occupancies of over 100 per cent (Hollander *et al.* 1990), psychiatric services in many inner-city areas are offering little apart from a 'madness and medicine' service. People are not kept in hospital long enough to benefit properly from treatment and are discharged at the first possible opportunity. Moreover, personal experience suggests that psychiatrists may well be reluctant to admit homeless people because they know that it will be difficult to discharge them to satisfactory accommodation.

## Discharge policies

As part of the 'stretched-service' scenario, it would appear that at least some patients are discharged without proper plans being made for them. In particular, psychiatrists have been criticized for discharging homeless patients to hostels or night-shelters rather than waiting until there is more appropriate accommodation available. This issue has been partially addressed by the section 117 provisions of the Mental Health Act, 1983, which require that a multidisciplinary meeting involving hospital staff, social workers and relatives be held prior to discharge to ensure an adequate treatment and support plan after discharge. However, it is obligatory only for those patients who have been detained under a section of the Act and takes no account of local deficiencies in services, whether in psychiatry, housing or social work. However, it may be unrealistic to expect catchment area psychiatrists to do otherwise when there are severely disturbed people almost literally queuing up to gain admission. In at least one London teaching hospital, several psychiatric wards have bed occupancies of over 100 per cent, with new admissions occupying a bed as soon as or before the previous occupant has been discharged (Neville and Masters 1991).

## Hostel issues

### Nature of direct access hostels

Users of direct access hostels do not have to be organized to receive the accommodation and help that the institution offers. As there is no very formal vetting system and hours of admission are usually very flexible, appointment keeping is not such a problem as it is with more discriminating services. Most offer a package of some sort of 'total support' involving shelter, food, clothing, help with benefits and eventually help with re-housing.

All these different needs are, to a greater or lesser extent, met from this one place; there is little co-ordination or travelling around that the resident has to do. A certain amount of advocacy and support will be taken on by hostel staff, although this sort of involvement may be found difficult due to a lack of understanding of the processes involved in mental illnesses. Overall, many direct access hostels have, or at least had, most of the characteristics of the old psychiatric hospitals. Both sorts of institution offered total care, albeit of a fairly low standard, and fostered institutionalization (Grunberg and Eagle 1990).

## Hostel closures

Altogether, nearly 7,000 direct access hostel beds have disappeared from the London scene over the last ten years. There were many reasons for this. The bulk of these beds were located in the large, squalid, Dickensian institutions that Orwell described so vividly in the 1930s, and which, quite frankly, had out-stayed their welcome. It was no longer acceptable for men and women to be accommodated in dormitories of fifty or a hundred beds with perhaps one lavatory and bath between them. It was no longer acceptable for hostel residents to be chucked out at 9 o'clock in the morning and left to roam the streets until the doors were opened again in the evening. It was no longer acceptable for inmates to be at the mercy of ill-paid, unsupervised and often corrupt hostel staff. It was no longer acceptable to herd together so many individuals with multiple health problems and thereby generate the spread of diseases such as tuberculosis. So, they were shut down one by one, either because they could not satisfy fire safety standards, because they were no longer commercially viable in an era of rising land values or because of central government policy. In many instances strenuous and successful efforts were made to rehouse those residents who had made the hostel their home.

## Nature of replacement schemes

However, most of the replacement schemes were set up as secondary or tertiary referral hostels which required referral and assessment procedures. The precise and multiple functions of direct access facilities were ignored, forgotten or simply not considered. This meant that many of those who would have used the old hostels became effectively excluded, most particularly those with long-term mental health problems.

It is therefore highly likely that the increasing numbers of homeless people on the streets have been generated primarily by the disappearance of direct access accommodation.

## Schizophrenia issues

Given that there is, and has been for some time, a large number of ex-psychiatric patients who become homeless, how is it that they accumulated in hostels which were originally intended for the travelling working man?

The marked disorganization of thought and action that often takes place during the course of a psychotic illness such as schizophrenia may make it very difficult for the individual to negotiate the long and complex procedures that are required to both gain access to housing and thereafter maintain it. Thus, those facilities which demand little in terms of motivation or organization on the part of an individual will be most likely to accumulate people with long-term mental illnesses. In specific relation to these illnesses, direct access hostels also exhibit two features that are strikingly reminiscent of the old mental hospitals:

1 The wide range of bizarre behaviours tolerated;
2 The general non-intrusiveness of other residents and staff.

These aspects of hostel life may well result in an emotional climate similar to those in which low 'expressed emotion' may reduce the likelihood of relapse and which may be subjectively comfortable for the schizophrenic (Leff and Vaughn 1981). However, the lack of appropriate stimulation means that no progress is made towards rehabilitation or resocialization (Wing and Brown 1970). Over the last thirty years, the result has been a dreary, demeaning status quo of perpetual dependence in a grim environment for the homeless person with schizophrenia.

## Access to housing

An American study (Alisky and Iczkowski 1990) has suggested that people with a mental health problem are discriminated against in the housing market. Even if symptoms are perfectly well controlled, their lack of money excludes them from the bulk of housing available for rent. In addition, landlords will choose not to let to those who mention a history of mental illness.

## BARRIERS TO SERVICE PROVISION

Having established that many people with long-term mental illness become homeless and lost to psychiatric services, how is it that they become alienated from the very services that are supposed to be offering them care?

## Institutional barriers

### Appointment systems

These are an important mechanism for ensuring that patients or clients do not have to wait unnecessarily and for maximizing the use of limited professional time. However, they tend to be institutional and ignore the fact that, to make use of clinics and appointments, one must have control over one's own time. Paradoxically, in spite of the lack of obvious conventional commitments, this is one thing the homeless person does not have to the same degree as the domiciled. Their use of time is determined by factors such as the unpredictability of waiting times at the DSS or homeless persons' unit or the opening hours of day centres and facilities where they can obtain free food, wash clothes and meet friends.

### Catchment areas

Most psychiatric services are now sectorized, meaning that a particular consultant team has responsibility for providing a service to a defined geographical area. Catchment areas are an important way of allocating professional responsibility for an individual and of ensuring continuing follow-up. However, an individual's right of access to such a service is determined by their address and, if they do not have one, it is difficult to get a service to take continued responsibility.

### Rigid working practices

Where treatment is concerned, in spite of many psychiatrists' insistence that the home is the best place to conduct an assessment, psychiatric services have tended to remain in institutions, albeit district general hospitals rather than asylums.

### Follow-up arrangements

In many instances the old adage 'No news is good news' seems to hold. When patients fail to turn up for appointments or do not open their doors to visiting community psychiatric nurses, they will often be dropped by the psychiatric service. In view of the limited resources available this may indeed make sense, but it also makes it much easier for people quietly to deteriorate and slip through the net. Psychiatric services are not alone in this as social workers are often encouraged to close long-standing cases to clear the decks for new and no doubt urgent ones.

## Community care

The inadequacy of the arrangements for care outside hospital for those with chronic mental illnesses has been commented on since the mid-1960s. In spite of this, very little thought seems to have been given to the issue until the last five years, when the disappearance of many psychiatric hospitals became imminent. Although psychiatric services may have deinstitutionalized themselves from the old asylums, they have often become reinstitutionalized in district general hospitals. The move from the asylums has coincided with psychiatric services abdicating any responsibility for social care, and this function has not yet been taken up by social service departments (Weller 1985).

More recently, the establishment of community mental health centres has been seen as a desirable move into the community for the psychiatric services. Unfortunately, the majority of the first wave of such establishments seem to have targeted better-functioning clients and neglected those with the more intractable and long-term mental illnesses (Sayce *et al.* 1991). Of course, it is precisely this latter group who are most likely to drift away from services and to become homeless.

## Inter-agency co-operation

The multiple needs of those with long-term mental illness mean that multiple agencies, health, social and housing, need to be involved in providing a comprehensive package of social care in addition to any specifically psychiatric input. Unfortunately, in many areas health and social services seem to be permanently at loggerheads and joint planning a pious hope for the future rather than a present reality.

## Communication

Even within agencies, poor communication is the norm rather than the exception. This encourages inappropriate prescribing by multiple GPs and hospital departments to a single client, with one professional not knowing what the other is doing. Again, we may find two or more housing departments involved, often ignorant of what their counterparts in another borough are doing.

## Philosophies of care

Inevitably, the different agencies involved have differing philosophies of care. For instance, most mental health services consider that individuals are unable to make informed choices when in the throes of a relapse of a severe mental illness. However, this view is not universally held. Many housing organizations take the view that people are always fully responsible for their choices and actions, no matter how thought disordered or deluded they may be. In my experience this attitude tends to produce inappropriate evictions, when a disturbed and often distressed client may be deemed, by his or her difficult behaviour, to have made a decision to act irresponsibly or anti-socially in breach of their tenancy agreement. To be fair, the inaccessibility of psychiatric help has often made it difficult for housing agencies to respond in any other way.

## Professional attitudes

Homeless agencies repeatedly report that their clients have been unable to register with GPs, have been treated in an offhand manner in hospitals or have been given the 'brush-off' in casualty departments. Doctors, nurses and receptionists are reprimanded and exhorted to do better but, by and large, little serious thought has been given to the reasons for this unprofessional behaviour on the part of men and women who regard themselves as professional and generally behave professionally in other respects and with other patients.

When one talks to either hospital staff or general practitioners, many express a considerable degree of therapeutic nihilism regarding the homeless. Some of this may indeed stem from bad experiences that staff may have had with homeless clients, often in casualty departments, but I believe there are other important factors to consider.

## Stereotyping

Professionals are not immune from holding the popular stereotypes of the homeless that pervade our culture. They tend therefore to perceive the homeless as being alcoholic, personality disordered, feckless, as having chosen to live in this way. This in turn means that they have very low expectations of homeless clients and that they may well not do as much for them as they would for domiciled patients.

## Multiple needs

Most professionals still work in an effectively mono-disciplinary environment. When they are confronted with a client who is both homeless and mentally ill, they are presented with a spectrum of multiple problems, most of which they do not have the skills to deal with. They may therefore experience profound feelings of impotence and feel that they actually have nothing to offer – 'What difference can I make?'

## Lack of a 'substrate for health'

Most medical and psychiatric staff are trained to examine fairly circumscribed areas of pathology. Their repertoire of interventions tends to assume the presence of the social factors (housing, adequate nutrition and a social network) that make possible health and, indeed, treatment. In the absence of these normative social frameworks, purely medical or psychiatric interventions may be perceived as pointless.

## Myth of mobility

This often seems to lead medical services to writing off the homeless client with 'He/she'll only move on to a different part of the country tomorrow, so what's the point in getting involved?' The old romantic myth of the homeless man as tramp, wandering the country with the seasons, clearly dies hard.

Taken together, these factors produce a therapeutic nihilism that not only prevents the professional from doing what they can, but may even serve as a conscious, or unconscious, justification for neglect.

### Lifestyle barriers

*Psychiatric treatment*

This tends to be low on a homeless person's list of priorities. Not surprisingly, the demands of securing basic survival needs such as food, shelter and money are often felt to be more pressing than appointments with doctors or nurses (Ball 1984).

## Poor access to services

The domiciled person who wishes to make use of psychiatric services will have his or her GP as both a guide to those services and an advocate with them. For the homeless person with no regular GP this is not the case, and any approaches tend to be made through casualty departments. For obvious reasons, their activities are orientated towards brief intervention rather than the continued involvement and advocacy that is necessary for continuity of care.

## Mobility

Mobility is as often forced upon the homeless as it is chosen. The reality is that, certainly in London, much of this mobility is relatively local. Unfortunately, you do not have to move very far to stray into another team's catchment area and thereby become their responsibility.

## Distrust of officialdom

To most (all?) official bodies, homeless people mean trouble because their predicament inevitably makes demands that they cannot meet. Hospitals and GPs are reluctant to take on the homeless and social security regulations seem especially designed to penalize them. Council housing departments are, in practice, only really interested in homeless families and those deemed vulnerable, as these are the only groups towards whom they have statutory responsibilities. The police as often as not are involved in moving on the homeless or arresting them for drunkenness. It is not surprising that the homeless should be suspicious and distrustful of any service that smacks of the institution or bureaucracy, as many generic psychiatric services still do.

## INTERVENTIONS

### General practice

Until recently, the homeless mentally ill were more likely to receive whatever mental health service they did from a general practitioner than from a psychiatrist. This perhaps resulted from the public health anxieties that were generated by the old hostels, particularly with regard to tuberculosis. It may therefore be helpful to look at some models of primary care provision that have emerged.

Sessional work has been done by district GPs in direct access hostels and day centres for the homeless. This has the virtue of establishing a local medical connection and the opportunity to register. However, in practice the work is usually limited both by the physical conditions pertaining and by the limited amount of time available to the doctor.

Specialist walk-in clinics, such as the one in Great Chapel Street in Soho, seem to be highly successful in opening up access to services for clients. They are located in the right place and – as one American psychiatrist has put it – they 'eschew many of the intake and assessment protocols that ritually confirm clienthood'. There is also a feeling that, as many potential clients are somewhat estranged from 'straight' society, the specialist nature of the service may be helpful – they do not have to compete with more obviously 'attractive' or easy clients.

One interesting supplement to this particular project is their 'sick-bay', a ten-bedded house for those who are too ill to be on the streets, but who are reluctant to go into hospital. Again, it is the non-institutional nature of this establishment that renders it acceptable and therefore of use. More recently a mobile clinic was established to serve the 'cardboard city' community underneath the South Bank complex in Waterloo, but this had to be abandoned following violence to staff.

More radically, in the absence of any reasonable GP service, nurse practitioner services have sprung up in one or two places where an experienced nurse has decided to offer a primary care service *faute de mieux* (*General Practitioner* 1987). These services have produced problems regarding prescribing and even legal difficulties. It was as a result of one of these pioneering nurses running into legal problems that the HHELP project in East London was set up. This was established as a multidisciplinary primary care service, involving nurses, social workers and alcohol workers as well as sessional GPs working with a variety of voluntary organizations.

## Psychiatry

Where have psychiatric services been all this time? The situation of being able to ignore the problem no longer holds, following the closure en masse of direct access hostels up and down the country and the subsequent rise of visible homelessness and, more particularly, of numerous disturbed individuals on the streets. A recent study revealed that 16 per cent of districts now have some sort of specialized health care provision for the homeless (Roderick *et al.* 1991).

Psychiatrists have and do offer sessions in direct access hostels and have run special out-patient clinics for the homeless, but these have been rather mono-professional efforts. Two psychiatrists now offer sessions to the Great Chapel Street clinic. A multidisciplinary walk-in service was set up in King's Cross, but seemed to attract a younger, less-disabled clientele.

In the US, numerous projects have sprung up. In New York, the 'Psychiatry Shelter Program' had a multidisciplinary psychiatric team working on site in hostels and shelters (Caton *et al.* 1990). They found that evaluation and subsequent client tracking were quite possible. Unfortunately, they found that their activities resulted in a higher rate of admission to hospital for their clients.

Another New York project focused at the point of discharge from hospital of homeless patients. A 'post-discharge residential programme' was set up using twenty-five rooms in an old flop-house which had been taken over by a supportive housing agency. A case-management approach was used and they found that they could support clients with very significant levels of psychopathology.

A more dramatic effort was the 'Project HELP Mobile Outreach Service' (Baxter and Hopper 1984), which seems to have consisted of an ambulance equipped with a crew of psychiatric personnel. They cruised the streets of New York waiting for emergency calls, whereupon they would swoop and do an assessment with a view to incarceration. To their credit, only 2 per cent of those assessed were actually detained. To my mind more significantly, they noted that prolonged intermittent contact resulted in engagement with even the least promising and most suspicious clients.

Two projects with a less specifically medical orientation were the LA 'Skid Row Mental Health Service' (Farr 1984) and the 'Community Living Room' (Segal and Baumohl 1985). Both offered a wide range of survival services, hanging-out space and psychiatric services.

An experiment rather closer in spirit to many of the American efforts was the Lewisham and North Southwark Psychiatric Team for Single Homeless People, set up in 1987 with a three-year DHSS grant (Brent Smith and Dean 1990). It was designed to provide a service to an area of South East London with 800 beds in traditional hostels and several day centres for the homeless. The size of this homeless population required a substantial commitment and so six full-time and two part-time posts were created, including medical, social work, housing and research staff. A multidisciplinary service was provided, working in the hostels themselves and later in day centres for the homeless. A controlled study conducted by this team suggested that, compared with an advice and co-ordinating model of service, a case-management approach was much more successful at engaging clients and sustaining contact with them.

## SERVICE STRATEGIES

Given the difficulties that exist, how can existing psychiatric services improve their performance in relation to homeless people?

### Finding a key worker

When treatment plans are started with homeless clients, they often fall apart because it is automatically assumed that there is no carer on the outside with whom contact can be maintained. For those with homes it would be a GP and homeless people often do not have a GP. However, there is nearly always a person or organization in some sort of caring role with whom they maintain contact and who should be informed. This might be a hostel or day-centre worker, an alcohol counsellor, a minister of religion, a social worker or a probation officer – the list is potentially endless. Of course, they will usually not be medical personnel and so issues of confidentiality may arise. These can be overcome by obtaining the client's written permission and/or by producing an edited version of documents such as discharge summaries.

### Flexibility

The conventional system of organizing access to a service by means of clinic times will not do for the homeless client. It is therefore desirable to negotiate times to meet the homeless client that fit in with their often irregular time-table, which may indeed change from week to week. If possible, users should be able, as and when necessary, to drop in.

### NFA rotas

Many psychiatric units, especially in large cities, have what they call an 'NFA rota'. This is a consultant rota which allocates to the consultants in turn clients of 'no fixed abode' who do not seem to belong to anybody's catchment area. Unfortunately, allocation in this way does not usually confer 'ownership' of the client and so if they present on a future occasion and another consultant is on the rota for that day, then they will be taken on by that consultant. And so nobody accepts continuing responsibility for the client and their care is unnecessarily fragmented. To improve continuity of care, allocation of a client via the NFA rota should confer continuing responsibility for them, even if on another occasion they should present when a different consultant is on duty for NFA clients.

### 'Homelessness' information

Professionals often find themselves hamstrung by their lack of knowledge of the facilities available locally to the homeless. These commonly include hostels, day centres, sources of cheap or free food and clothing, alcohol counselling services and advice centres. Each health authority or trust should obtain or create a directory of these services that is concise enough to be of use in a busy ward, general practice, or casualty department (*Homelessness Handbook* 1988).

### Prescribing

Abusable drugs should not be prescribed. Although most of the recipients use their medication responsibly, it should not be forgotten that drugs such as the benzodiazepines, heminevrin and procyclidine have a not inconsiderable street value. In circumstances where it may be impossible to get hold of money any other way, it may be very tempting to sell off part of one's prescription.

### THE FUTURE

These London services are old hat by American standards. Nevertheless, they are seen as useful innovations in service provision to a demonstrably needy and under-served client group which has become more obviously visible over the last few years. However, there is considerable anxiety that provision of specialist services in this way will, whatever the direct benefits to individuals, serve only to marginalize the homeless further. There are certainly difficulties in providing an acceptable service to the homeless through existing generic services, but this argues as much for modifying existing practices as it does for establishing entirely new services.

So, what are the ways in which these specialist services are able to out-perform generic psychiatric services? Experience suggests that they engage those patients/clients that standard services do not because they are:

'Out there'
Informal
Flexible
Dealing with social needs as well as psychiatric ones
Multidisciplinary
Collaborative
Responsive to changing circumstances.

But these principles should characterize any desirable community psychiatric service. They are directly applicable to the practice of general psychiatry in the non-institutional era. It may be said that homelessness is an extreme predicament, that the responses it generates are unique to this situation and cannot be generalized. An extreme it may be, but it is an extremity of a continuum, the social continuum of poverty and deprivation, and the homeless are merely at one end of this continuum. The extremity of their situation brings sharply into focus issues which affect *all* clients of psychiatric services with long-term mental illnesses, as most, if not actually homeless, are certainly some way down that social continuum.

So, 'homelessness psychiatry' should not be seen as a micro-speciality in its own right, but as one end of the current spectrum of community care. I would go further and say that it is a model for the future of psychiatry as it applies to chronic mental illness in the community. The aim for the future surely has to be the establishment of community services that serve the entire community and take into account the special needs of disadvantaged minority groups.

How is this to be achieved? A first step must be to establish a single authority responsible for community care. At present health services and housing/social services have their goals and priorities set by authorities that are completely independent of each other. Even with joint-planning exercises, this makes it almost impossible to construct seamless packages of care that include both psychiatric and social provision. There has been talk of a 'Minister for Community Care', but this authority would probably be most effective at the level of the new purchasing authorities (Ashley-Miller 1990).

Psychiatric services must be prepared to provide their service across catchment area boundaries to a much greater extent than they do at present. This could be in the form of a continuing care team that would cover several districts, as happens with existing homelessness services. However, the ramshackle information systems that at present pervade the NHS are not up to the job. In order to keep track of people who move across our artificial boundaries, computerized case registers need to be established. These will, however, demand a considerable investment in time, effort and training if they are to be clinically effective and not merely tools for the health service accountants.

Lastly, psychiatrists in training should spend far less of their time in hospitals. In general medicine, medical student training is beginning to move from teaching hospitals to general practices, where most medical activity takes place. Similarly, in many areas it is voluntary sector agencies who provide the bulk of care outside hospital. It is in these settings that the psychiatrists of tomorrow should be spending more of their time as these are the places where people's real lives are lived.

# REFERENCES

Alisky, J.M. and Iczkowski, K.A. (1990) 'Barriers to housing for deinstitutionalised psychiatric patients', *Hospital and Community Psychiatry* 41: 93–5.

Allderidge, P. (1979) 'Hospitals, madhouses and asylums: cycles in the care of the insane', *British Journal of Psychiatry* 134: 321–34.

Anderson, N. (1923) *The Hobo: The Sociology of the Homeless Man*, Chicago: University of Chicago Press.

Appleby, L. (1985) 'Documenting the relationship between homelessness and psychiatric hospitalisation', *Hospital and Community Psychiatry* 36: 732–7.

Ashley-Miller, A. (1990) 'Community care – research studies are essential', *British Medical Journal*, 300: 487.

Ball, J. (1984) 'A survey of the problems and needs of homeless consumers of acute psychiatric services', *Hospital and Community Psychiatry* 35: 917–21.

Bassuk, E.L. (1984) 'The homelessness problem', *Scientific American* 251: 28–33.

Baxter, B. and Hopper, K. (1984) 'Shelter and housing for the homeless mentally ill', in R. Lamb (ed.) *The Homeless Mentally Ill*, Washington, DC: American Psychiatric Association.

Becker, T. (1985) 'Psychiatric reform in Italy – how does it work in Piedmont?' *British Journal of Psychiatry* 147: 254–60.

Berry, C. and Orwin, A. (1966) 'No fixed abode: a survey of mental hospital admissions', *British Journal of Psychiatry* 112: 1019–25.

Bogue, D.J. (1963) *Skid Row in American Cities*, Community & Family Study Centre, University of Chicago, pp. 482–3.

Brent Smith, H. and Dean, R. (1990) *Plugging the Gaps*, London: Lewisham and North Southwark Health Authority.

Caton, C.L.M., Wyatt, R.J. Grunberg, J. and Felix, A. (1990) 'An evaluation of a mental health program for homeless men', *Psychiatry*, 147(3): 286–9.

Edwards, G., Williamson, V., Hawker, A., Hensman, C. and Postsyan, S. (1968) 'Census of a reception centre', *British Journal of Psychiatry* 114: 1031–9.

Faris, R.E. and Dunham, H.W. (1939) *Mental Disorders in Urban Areas: An Ecological Study of Schizophrenia and Other Psychoses*, Chicago: University of Chicago Press.

Farr, K. (1984) 'A mental health treatment program for the homeless mentally ill in the Los Angeles skid row area', in B.E. Jones (ed.) *Treating The Homeless: Urban Psychiatry's Challenge*, Washington, DC: American Psychiatric Press pp. 65–92.

*General Practitioner* (1987) 'Expect some harsh words from Sister Barbara'.

Grunberg, J. and Eagle, P.F. (1990) 'Shelterization: how the homeless adapt to shelter living', *Hospital and Community Psychiatry* 41: 521–5.

Gunn, J. (1974) 'Prisons, shelters, and homeless men', *Psychiatric Quarterly*, 48: 505–12.

Herzberg, J.L. (1987) 'No fixed abode: a comparison of men and women admitted to an East London psychiatric hospital', *British Journal of Psychiatry* 150: 621–7.

Hollander, D., Tobiansky, R. and Powell, R. (1990) 'Crisis in admission beds', *British Medical Journal* 301: 664.

*Homelessness Handbook* (1988) Psychiatric Team for Single Homeless People, Lewisham and North Southwark Authority.

Lamb, R.H. (1984) 'Deinstitutionalisation and the homeless mentally ill', *Hospital and Community Psychiatry* 35: 899–907.

Leff, J. and Vaughn, C. (1981) 'The role of maintenance therapy and relatives' expressed emotion in relapse of schizophrenia: a two-year follow up', *British Journal of Psychiatry* 139: 102–4.

Lodge Patch, I. (1971) 'Homeless men in London: demographic findings in a lodging house sample', *British Journal of Psychiatry* 118: 313–17.

Marshall, M. (1989) 'Collected and neglected: are Oxford hostels for the homeless filling up with disabled psychiatric patients?', *British Medical Journal* 299: 706–8.

Mental Health Act 1983, London: HMSO, chapter 20.

Neville, M. and Masters, D. (1991) *A Report of In-patient Activity on Mental Illness Wards at Guy's Hospital for the Full Year 1990*, Lewisham & North Southwark Mental Health Executive.

*NHS Hospital Administrative Statistics: Health and Personal Social Services Statistics for England* (1990). London: Department of Health.

Orwell, G. (1933) *Down and Out in Paris and London*, London: Penguin.

Priest, R.G. (1971) 'The homeless person and the psychiatric services: an Edinburgh survey', *British Journal of Psychiatry* 128: 128–36.

Roderick, R., Victor, C. and Connelly, J. (1991) 'Is housing a public health issue? A survey of directors of public health', *British Medical Journal* 302: 157–60.

Sayce, L., Craig, T.K.J. and Boardman, A.P. (1991) 'The development of Community Mental Health Centres in the U.K.', *Social Psychiatry and Psychiatric Epidemiology* 26: 14–20.

Segal, S.P. and Baumohl, J. (1985) 'The community living room', *Social Casework: The Journal of Contemporary Social Work* February: 111–16.

Tidmarsh, D. and Wood, S. (1972) 'Psychiatric aspects of destitution: a study of the Camberwell reception centre', in J. Wing and A.M. Hailey (eds) *Evaluating a Community Psychiatric Service*, Oxford: Oxford University Press, pp. 327–46.

Timms, P.W. and Fry, A.H. (1989) 'Homelessness and mental illness', *Health Trends* 21: 70–1.

Vexliard, A. (1957) *Le Clochard: Etude de psychologie sociale*, Paris: Desclee de Brower.

Weller, M. (1985) 'Friern Hospital: where have all the patients gone?', *Lancet* 1: 569–71.

Weller, M. (1986) 'Health care in a destitute population: Christmas 1985', *Bulletin of the Royal College of Psychiatrists*, 10: 233–5.

Whiteley, J.S. (1955) 'Down and out in London: mental illness in the lower social groups', *Lancet* 2: 608–10.

Wilmanns, K. (1906) *Zur Psychopathologie des Landstreichers: Eine Klinische Studie*, Leipzig: Barth.

Wing, J.K. and Brown, G.W. (1970) *Institutionalism and Schizophrenia*, London: Cambridge University Press.

# 5    Alcohol and single homelessness
## An outreach approach

*Lynda Freimanis*

## INTRODUCTION

There is a certain inevitability that in a book about homelessness one chapter would focus on alcohol use. A variety of studies in both Britain and America have agreed that approximately a third of people living on the streets experience significant and on-going problems with alcohol.

The purpose of this chapter is not to review or to add to these findings. Academic research on vagrancy or the incidence of 'alcoholism' in the skid row population has done little to address the problem. Rather, this chapter attempts to outline a pragmatic and co-ordinated response to the alcohol problems experienced by individuals in the single homeless community.

A discussion about alcohol and homelessness evokes certain stereotypes: 'homeless drinker', 'the vagrant alcoholic', 'the derelict', 'the skid row dosser' and 'the jake drinker'. Society has clearly labelled its victims. Yet the causal link between the use of alcohol and homelessness is arguable. The usefulness of the debate to the drinkers on the street is also questionable as it does little to enhance, empower or render agencies more accessible to their needs.

In the eighteenth century alcohol was generally viewed as a positive and healthy part of life, the exception being the drinking of gin by the destitute population of London which was perceived as a social evil necessitating a central government response. Society continues to hold an ambivalent attitude towards alcohol. The use of alcohol may be accepted behind closed doors but it is certainly not acceptable when it is taken out on to the streets. The context of their drinking therefore renders the street population visible and, thus, vulnerable to scapegoating. This is regardless of the fact that their actual alcohol intake may often be less than that of their counterparts in the housed population. Intoxication, it would appear, is a privilege accorded only to those who have a house to become drunk in.

Individuals experiencing problems with alcohol are on the streets or hostel circuit for a whole variety of reasons. These may include anything from marriage break-up, unemployment, emotional crisis, discharge from the armed forces or running away from an intolerable home situation. Although there may be an academic need to ascertain the reasons behind a homeless person's drinking, it is more relevant to focus on how that individual might survive more safely. They can then be encouraged to take positive steps towards change when the time is right for them.

A focus on individual need is an important first step in truly addressing the needs of the homeless street drinker. Yet progress is restrained by both the stereotypes constructed by society and the caring profession's insatiable need for facts.

Men and women struggling with the problems of alcohol and who live on the streets or in hostels are entitled to a range of options and a coherent service to meet their needs. The context in which these needs are expressed has tended to provoke a judgemental and punitive response. A breakthrough in the provision of services for the drinking homeless can be achieved only if stereotypes are constantly challenged and confronted.

Considerable progress has been made in the field of alcohol and homelessness since the 'inebriate asylums' of the nineteenth and early twentieth centuries. It is difficult, however, to assess how close the caring professions are now to addressing the complex and individual needs of the homeless street drinker. Future progress lies in the marshalling of skills and resources to provide a unified response. Agencies and professionals from both the voluntary and state sectors need to recognize and utilize the existing community-based resources. This would reduce the isolation experienced by single homeless drinkers and more effectively integrate the individual into the community.

## AN OUTREACH SERVICE

In 1990 the Drink Crisis Centre initiated an outreach service for the street drinking population. Funded by the Department of Health, the brief of the workers was to bridge the gap between the street drinking population and the existing alcohol service provision. The experience of the community alcohol worker at the East London Homeless Health Project (HHELP) has demonstrated the impact of an outreach provision. Within the space of nine months over eight hundred contacts had been made with men and women experiencing difficulties with alcohol in their lives. The majority of these individuals had consistently failed to access services relevant to their needs.

Although part of the multidisciplinary team, the HHELP community alcohol worker had experienced isolation while inundated with individuals presenting complex problems. From its inception the Drink Crisis Centre outreach team attempted to work with other professionals and agencies already engaged in the field of alcohol and homelessness, thus avoiding the dual problems of lack of co-ordination and worker isolation.

In attempting to achieve a co-ordinated and coherent response the outreach team was aware the alcohol field comprised a number of disparate agencies often working in isolation. This created specialized and exclusive responses reflecting the belief systems and philosophies of the agency rather than addressing the clients' needs. Clearly this is detrimental to those who require help from alcohol services.

## SHORT-TERM GOALS

The short-term goals for the DCC outreach team were:

*To contact agencies and professionals working in the fields of alcohol and homelessness with a view to working towards developing a cohesive network of service provision*

The team saw that working together with existing agencies was the way forward and particular emphasis was placed on achieving common goals. Co-operation with existing agencies enabled the adoption of a pragmatic response which avoided conflict with established modes of practice.

*To offer a street service directly to men and women who are homeless and experiencing problems with alcohol in their lives*

From the conception of the team a commitment to a target client group was identified: homeless men and women experiencing alcohol problems. It was recognized that, during the daily experience of working on the streets, contact with other client groups would occur. Therefore there was a need to acknowledge limitations and clearly focus the team's energy on individuals experiencing problems with alcohol. Individuals with other needs were referred to specialized agencies as and when necessary, thus avoiding the tendency to work with clients whom it was more appropriate to refer on to more relevant services.

### To become a familiar aspect of the street community and to engender a mutual attitude of respect and trust

Obviously it was inappropriate that workers should become truly part of the community. However, using social work skills of genuineness, empathy and active listening, it was hoped that relationships could be forged within the clients' territory. A clear distinction was insisted upon between empathy and sympathy. The emphasis was on empathy, which encourages empowerment, enabling a client to make changes or to cope better within their environment. A genuine attempt was made to work at the client's own pace toward attainable goals, thus avoiding the social work trap of workers 'feeling the need' to change a client's situation before the client was ready.

### To work alongside existing 'outreach services' in an attempt to improve access to existing service provision

Homeless street drinkers have a very low profile with many of the 'helping agencies'; this is particularly true of casualty departments and social services. This is also evident, though more subtle, in the voluntary sector. By making contact with a large, diverse group of agencies including day-centre workers, hostel workers and primary health care teams, the project attempted to encourage them to work with, rather than avoid, homeless clients with alcohol problems. The team also wanted to confront prevailing attitudes to homeless street drinkers within the helping professions. This highlighted the need for training and consultancy on an on-going basis.

### Where appropriate to refer and to escort clients to appropriate service provisions and thus to facilitate the transition from the street culture into the new setting

The outreach team retained a client's case while they went through admission and acceptance into a new provision. Without undermining the skill of the client this additional support was considered important for two reasons. First, transition and change are difficult experiences to deal with per se and a form of continuity of care for an individual is important. Second, the firsthand exchange of information from one set of professionals to the receiving group is an essential step in inter-agency co-operation and support. The nature and length of the involvement of the outreach team with the receiving agency was dictated by the needs of the individual. The role of the outreach worker could be seen primarily as one of enabling or enhancing rather than 'minding'. For the long-term street drinker to move to the Drink Crisis Centre or a dry house can be a massive step necessitating appropriate professional support. Bridging the gap between the street drinking environment and mainstream provision demands that the client has support, not only to move physically from the street, but also with their effort to overcome psychological barriers to a non-alcohol-dependent lifestyle.

*To challenge and confront attitudes and stereotypes held by individuals and agencies, in the belief that these attitudes further stigmatize and marginalize women and men who are homeless and have alcohol problems*

This is an on-going aim. It is both integral to the approach taken by the team and requires the adoption of an advocacy role on the client's behalf.

## A MODEL OF CHANGE

In order to translate these goals into practice the team sought to develop a model of change which could be used in the context of streetwork. The model is based on the work of Procashka and DiClemente. Briefly the model is as follows:

Pre-contemplation: the stage where the individual has not considered change as necessary.

Contemplation: the individual is in a stage of raised awareness of the negative consequences of the behaviour and is contemplating change as a result.

Action: the person engages in efforts to bring about change.

Maintenance: the person retains the changes made.

Relapse: the person resumes the old behaviour. It is important to the model to consider relapse as part of the cycle. Studies have found that, while 70–80 per cent of people relapse, 84 per cent of these return to contemplation of change and so may learn to change by passing through the cycle several times.

A starting point is to build a relationship of mutual respect and mutual trust. The client needs to feel that the worker is genuine and is committed to working at the client's pace and in a way that respects the client's choice. An underlying belief that the client is a responsible adult capable of making responsible decisions and arriving at the right solution is fundamental to this approach, with the worker acting as a resource to this process by providing options, feedback, information and alternatives. The overall aims then are to:

a) Increase the client's self-esteem.
b) Increase the client's self-determination – to raise the person's own perception of their ability to engage in active and effective coping strategies.
c) To help the client to see any links between problems they readily acknowledge, i.e. health problems, difficulty in maintaining accommodation, accidents, etc., with drinking.
d) To provide accessible and relevant alternatives to the present drinking behaviour.

During the initial planning stage two key themes emerged. These could be broadly described as access and immediacy.


## ACCESS

The Drink Crisis Centre opened its doors in 1990 followed by the Rugby House Project. These two provisions endeavoured to alleviate the problems experienced by clients attempting to utilize services. Access to provisions for single homeless drinkers is fraught with difficulties and, although these projects have to some extent altered the situation, the demand for services remains high. While more facilities are not necessarily the answer, a greater understanding and flexibility is required from those services already in operation.

Before the onset of outreach initiatives, alcohol agencies made it nearly impossible for single homeless people to use their service. This proved especially so in the case of clients who needed a detoxification facility. Access had to be negotiated and renegotiated; criteria had to be met and clients were consistently found to be inappropriate. The drinker had to have no history of mental health problems nor a significant criminal record. Also they would be expected to make a complete break with their past lives. On occasions clients would be interviewed for a project, called back for a second interview, only then to be informed that they were unsuitable or being manipulative.

The criteria for the admission of single homeless men were extremely difficult to meet. For single women the picture was even bleaker. Before 1989 there were no residential community-based detoxification facilities in London for women. The only services available were hospital based. There were also isolated beds in psychiatric or general medical wards, neither of which could be described as conducive to a positive experience of detoxification. Beyond the criteria for admission the expectations that many of the agencies held were both unrealistic and exclusive. It was an unrealistic expectation that the clients would be on time for their appointments, given that they could not afford public transport, were sleeping out and had little access to telephones. The professional cynic has been heard to reply that the client was 'on time for the off-licence' or 'if they really wanted to detox. they would have been on time'. The element of truth in these comments is negated by the lack of understanding of the notion of 'future time' for a homeless person on the street.

Once accepted into a provision, clients often met unrealistic expectations from workers. They had to be motivated and not under the influence of any other medication (even if that medication had been provided by a GP), sober, willing to participate in religious activities and amenable to talking honestly about their past lives in large groups composed of people they had only recently met. Their continued accommodation was reliant on them staying dry. If they relapsed, a classic feature of alcohol dependency syndrome, they were asked to leave regardless of the period of time they had managed to remain sober. Sometimes attempts were made to provide alternative accommodation. The reality for many was a return to the streets more resentful, rejected and perceiving themselves to be a greater failure than when they first entered the facility.

The sense of failure and shame experienced by clients delayed future contemplation of change. The shop-front approach of the Alcohol Recovery Project alleviated to some extent the 'revolving door' pattern, yet it could still take months to encourage a client back into a provision. Relapses were rarely looked at positively or as an opportunity to work towards longer-term sobriety. Several episodes of relapse resulted in a client being labelled difficult, manipulative or beyond the reach of services.

Only the fellowship of Alcoholics Anonymous remained open to all. However, it has no residential component and has for some a rather highly developed spiritual approach. Alcoholics Anonymous can be useful once the individual has come off the streets and has a base, but it is extremely difficult to stay sober on the streets even if a regular AA attender.

## IMMEDIACY

The DCC outreach team emphasized the importance of providing an immediate practical response relevant to the individual's need. In any street session many of the individuals would be what Procashka and DiClemente termed pre-contemplators. They are not at the stage of wanting to change their situation. However, within each session there will be clients who are ready to move from contemplation to action. Delaying that action could mean that the person becomes disillusioned and decides that it is not worth the effort: moving back into pre-contemplation. The action necessary may be one of a whole range of options. A vulnerable, elderly man may need to move into a long-stay hostel, a young runaway to be put in contact with a more relevant service or an individual be given support and encouragement in the decision that their drinking problems need to be addressed. Whatever the window of opportunity in an individual's life, the relevant intervention needs to be made immediately, before the window closes.

The outreach team has often been able to respond immediately to the need for hostel accommodation. This has been achieved through the team's links with a variety of hostels and agencies in Central London. Until recently, if a detoxification placement was required, immediate action was thwarted by the problems of accessibility. Only the Drink Crisis Centre offered a twenty-four-hour service; Booth House in Whitechapel and Rugby House admit people only during office hours. It was impossible to get access to a detox. bed outside office hours if the Drink Crisis Centre was full.

In an attempt to address the problems of accessibility a network of holding beds has been established among hostels in Central London.

This 'holding network' means that individuals can be settled in a bed at night, monitored by hostel staff and then moved into one of three community detox. provisions within twenty-four hours. The outreach team facilitates the process and liaises with hostel workers in order to effect the move from hostel into detox. Thus the opportunity to make a useful intervention is not lost and the process of clients being turned away not to return for a week, if ever, has been interrupted.

Liaison with hostel workers has ensured that the problems of alcohol abuse have become dynamic rather than reactive items on hostel agendas – so much so that workers are now making appropriate referrals to various detox. provisions. So, encouraging progress is being made through close liaison with and utilizing of existing community-based resources.

The majority of individuals encountered during an outreach session do not want to stop drinking or leave the street. They want a brief chat, advice or information. The aim therefore is to use the continued contact with the client in order to facilitate the step from contemplation of change to change. Becoming part of the community scene essentially means being consistent, 'being there' as arranged. The outreach team quickly became part of the street network, so much so that known clients of the outreach team have brought new clients to the service.

## SETTING UP THE SERVICE

Before the formation of the Drink Crisis Centre outreach team there was no outreach provision which concentrated on people experiencing alcohol problems. Most of the outreach work focused on housing and drug-related problems. Therefore the project was breaking important new ground.

For the first two months, before the commencement of street work, the outreach team undertook an extensive tour of Central London agencies to become familiar with the services available to men and women who had alcohol problems and were street homeless. Many agencies continue to be visited on a regular basis to re-establish links, make new contracts and to ensure as far as possible that the outreach team is fully aware of the resources available in the community. Information given to clients on the street is therefore both relevant and accurate.

The agency visits had several functions. First, they enabled the team to experience at firsthand the nature and range of current service provision by meeting both the service providers and the grass-roots workers. Also much was learned from experiences of projects such as Thames Reach concerning the development of a street-based service.

Second, by visiting the agencies a platform was provided from which the work of the DCC and the role of the outreach team could be disseminated. Within the alcohol field outreach work had previously been confined to a 'shop-front' service. The suggestion of a literal outreach provision initiated much discussion and comment from the agencies all of which effectively contributed to the development of the project.

The significance of working within the street drinking community as a way of building up contacts between team members and individual drinkers had been demonstrated by the work of Thames Reach. Contact built up over weeks and months with the outreach team would hopefully enable the client to feel that he or she could use the service.

The outreach team sought to develop a more credible identity by meeting street drinkers within their own community. Workers were thus perceived as having an awareness of the problems individual drinkers faced in their day to day lives and were then in a better position to offer an accurate and relevant response to clients' needs.

Above all, it was clear to those involved in the outreach project that it was essential to use the services already in the community rather than creating specialist provisions.

Interest was expressed by most of the agencies visited; however, there were also a number of reservations and even some derision. It became obvious that the work of the outreach team would have greater impact on some agencies than others. Useful comments were expressed by agencies who targeted their services towards the needs of young people. The traditional dry house settings were seen to have little to offer a young person drinking destructively who had not developed a chronic pattern of consumption. This sort of feedback was extremely important and needs to be responded to by the alcohol field.

Workers involved with young street drinkers have encountered young people who have been using alcohol since the age of 12 or even younger. Resources clearly need to be focused to deal with the specific problem of young drinkers before patterns of alcohol dependency become ingrained. It is particularly important that a young person, perhaps reasonably new to the circuit, does not become caught in the 'revolving door' of failure and rejection, becoming part of a fringe group existing on the edge of society.

In response to those concerns the outreach team agreed to offer a consultancy service to agencies working with young drinkers. The team also became involved in providing training for their staff teams to allow them to work more effectively.

Agencies working in the field of housing and resettlement, although expressing interest in the concept of the Drink Crisis Centre, also voiced reservations about the link between housing and alcohol treatment and the rehabilitation process – the traditional 'dry house' model links housing with rehabilitation. An individual's secure housing status is therefore dependent on them staying dry. It cannot be considered a good use of resources or a positive therapeutic model to take a person from the street into a dry house where episodes or even one episode of drinking leads the individual to be evicted back onto the street or into a large traditional hostel. However, as Tim Cook in his description of the setting up of Rathcook demonstrated, it is extremely difficult to contain episodes of drinking in a residential setting where the general goal is to stay dry (Cook 1975). Similar situations have arisen in other projects which operate a 'relapse management' policy. Most often when clients have started drinking in the project premises they have either ended up wandering off or they have been evicted back onto the streets. It would be more realistic for the housing and the alcohol components to be kept separate. The alcohol agency could then offer a day programme or counselling outside the residential facility.

An insidious repercussion of linking accommodation with rehabilitation is that in various projects clients are staying dry until they are placed in accommodation. Once that goal is achieved they fail ferociously and in a short space of time they are quickly drawn back onto the streets. Again this reinforces a person's low self-esteem and the sense of being a failure. The answer lies in professionals working with clients to form plans of action focused on a reasonable goal, which encourages resettlement, life skills and work on alcohol problems.

The resettlement workers at St Botolph's crypt operate a more dynamic approach to homeless street drinkers. An attempt is made to resettle a person before they have really tackled their drinking problem. The theory behind this approach is that once the individual has a base to work from it is more likely that they might be able to address their drinking problems. Also, once housed, it is relatively easy to put them in touch with services. If their drinking gets seriously out of hand, detox. centres are available for drying out and they can then return to their own accommodation. To some extent this prevents the 'revolving door' syndrome and is arguably more cost-effective than continually referring people in and out of high-care hostel accommodation. However, this approach demands a more sophisticated and creative level of input by workers involved in its implementation. As with any approach, this model has worked for some clients and has been ineffective for others.

Joint work between alcohol workers and other professionals can be used beneficially in a variety of ways. An outreach alcohol worker can work in conjunction with an HIV/AIDS specialist or with a mental health worker where assessment is needed in order to ascertain the extent to which the problems experienced are due to alcohol or an underlying mental health problem.

Joint care plans within the luxury of a multidisciplinary team are both dynamic and common sense. However, when liaison is necessary by individuals within a variety of agencies, joint plans are not easily formed. It takes considerable perseverance and trust to establish a multidisciplinary care plan across agencies. Traditionally communications within the voluntary sector are based upon individual contacts and relationships rather than a management-led initiative. Recognition of the importance of liaison by voluntary section managers is a vital part of providing integrated services for clients.

## OFFERING THE SERVICE

Having established the need for an outreach service and identified the target group the decision was taken to offer the service in two distinct ways.

### The street service

Given the numerical limitations of the outreach team it was logical for the project to work with agencies already operating at a street level. Initially this took the form of joint work with workers from both the Bondway and the Rugby House Mobile Alcohol team. More sophisticated links were forged with Thames Reach and St Botolph's Crypt Resettlement Team.

This blend of agencies provided a more useful and effective response to the problems of single homeless drinkers. The core outreach team was extended and enabled to provide a more extensive service. The resources of these agencies were made available and accessible to the client group. In addition, the workers involved avoided the problem of isolation because they felt part of an integrated and supportive response. Finally, by developing a unified strategy these agencies were able to make a greater impact on the wider political scene. As a result they were able to raise the profile of the single homeless drinker who has tended to be ignored when resources are allocated.

### The timing of the service

After due thought and acknowledgement of the resources available, it was decided to offer the outreach service regularly in the early mornings and evenings. The team felt these were the times most relevant to the client group many of whom use day-centre provision during the day. A considerable gap in the service exists at the weekends but, because of staffing resources, the outreach team could not address that need.

Evenings were the obvious time for the outreach workers to focus their efforts. As day centres closed the client group gradually drifted back to their shelters or 'bashes'. The experience of Thames Reach had shown that it was possible to make contact with large numbers of people on the street in the evening. The outreach team were aware of several large drinking 'schools' where they could offer their service and also a network of soup runs offering the opportunity of contacting fairly large numbers of people in a relatively safe environment. As no other alcohol agency provided an evening service the outreach team was in an ideal position to make initial contact and then refer on to day-time provisions such as shop-fronts. Additionally the Drink Crisis Centre had evening vacancies because it offered a twenty-four-hour service.

Early mornings addressed another gap in the service to homeless drinkers. Prior to the outreach project only the Passage Day Centre in Victoria and the Webber Street Mission in Lambeth regularly offered a service before day centres opened their doors around ten o'clock. Therefore a number of contacts could be made while clients waited for services to open. Early morning was the most likely time to find street drinkers in a relatively sober state which was a definite advantage. Also the 'morning after' is a particularly painful time for heavy drinkers and they are therefore more likely to seek help.

The outreach project established a working pattern of two early mornings from six-thirty until ten-thirty and two evenings from seven until about midnight depending on the number of contacts.

**Where do we go?**

In order to encounter the largest number of clients, the outreach project focused its efforts in areas where they were guaranteed to meet street drinkers, thus ensuring the service would be available to as many people as possible. A regular pattern of street work was also established in order that people were aware of where the outreach workers were likely to be. This was considered a more effective use of resources than haphazardly attempting to meet need when and where it arose. Essentially the outreach workers offered a flexible response and regularly followed up referrals made by other teams. This flexible approach sometimes meant that arrangements and locations for work had to be changed. In these cases the outreach team attempted to notify the clients via the soup runs or workers in other agencies. Clients were therefore made aware that the team were involved in work elsewhere and had not simply absented themselves, communication and consistency being central to a trusting relationship. Positive involvement with workers in the helping professions or social services is unusual for individuals in the street community. They are commonly forgotten, left until last or let down. These experiences have constructed a barrier which needs to be met with common courtesy and the recognition of the need for good communication. A failure to meet client expectations can lead to workers being labelled as unreliable or uncooperative. Such labels are identical to those imposed, by members of the helping professions, on this client group.

The areas visited regularly by the outreach team were: Lincoln's Inn Fields, Kingsway, the Strand, the Temple Gardens and the area around the Embankment Tube. South of the river the team included Waterloo where they visited St John's Crypt steps, the 'Bullring' and the 'Hole in the Wall', an old and well-established street drinking area and one of the most Dickensian spots in modern London. Each of these venues provided valuable points of contact for the outreach workers to meet drinkers.

The early morning visits included Lincoln's Inn Fields, Temple Gardens and also early morning forays to early opening public houses surrounding the Bermondsey street market, Keyworth House DSS in Southwark, where many people who are NFA sign on, Finsbury Park, Camden Town and the area around the American Church in Tottenham Court Road where there is a regular school of Scots drinkers.

**Who goes there?**

The street work sessions are undertaken by pairs of workers. In the evening the ideal team consists of a male and a female worker where possible, otherwise two male workers. Two female workers was an acceptable morning team but, for safety reasons, was not acceptable during the evening. However, during the first year of operating there were only a few occasions when members of the team found themselves in threatening situations. Physical and verbal violence are an undeniable aspect of the street scene and so safety of workers is a high priority.

On almost every session the worker pairing consists of workers from different agencies: a Bondway Shelter worker alongside a Drink Crisis Centre worker or a Thames Reach worker with a Rugby House Mobile Alcohol Service worker. This model is surprisingly easy to effect, not least because all the workers involved are committed to providing the best possible service to the client group. By going beyond rigid allegiances to individual agencies the response to the problems of the drinking homeless is enhanced. This is particularly remarkable at a time when the voluntary sector is faced with the looming 'contract culture' and individual agencies are fighting for their own survival.

## Transport

The outreach team at the Drink Crisis Centre has at its disposal a black cab. This is used by the team to facilitate the admission of clients, especially in the evenings, into service provision. It proves to be particularly useful if the client is intoxicated or has problems with mobility. Furthermore, the cab is spacious enough for a worker to accompany a client and assist them if they are physically unwell.

The anonymity of the black cab in Central London also minimizes the chance that dissatisfied users might direct their wrath at the outreach team's transport. Its anonymity also means that clients can be escorted in privacy, with dignity and a measure of comfort, to the relevant service.

The black cab was the object of much ridicule when it was first considered as a means of transporting clients to the centres. Even the project leader expressed scepticism regarding the necessity of the vehicle. However, the cab proved its usefulness and regularly takes clients, swiftly and safely, to a variety of destinations.

## How do we keep in touch?

To encourage efficient communication with the outreach team's base and emergency services a mobile telephone is used. The mobile telephone is used regularly to make referrals to the centres and keep in contact with the base, notifying co-workers of delays or possible problems. By using a mobile telephone, liaison with other agencies is simplified. One disadvantage is that clients occasionally suspect that the telephone is being used to 'check them out'.

## Whom have we contacted?

The 'outreach' street sessions have led to many hundreds of contacts with street drinkers. Over a hundred of these contacts resulted in the individual being taken directly back to the Drink Crisis Centre for a stay of between one night and four weeks, after which they would have gone either into further treatment or to a hostel or other short-stay accommodation. Others have left, gone drinking and returned to the street. The team has kept in contact with them in the belief that work of this type is long term and rarely 'successful' on the first attempt.

Over twenty have gone into Rugby House in North London and Bondway has accepted over a hundred referrals. These have mostly been older, extremely vulnerable men, who are long-term street dwellers with physical or mental health problems. Some of them have then been referred on to the Drink Crisis Centre, Rugby House or Booth House, while others have moved from short-stay to longer-stay accommodation.

The team have encountered a variety of people who defy any stereotype that exists about single homeless drinkers. Young women and old men, people who have only been out for a few nights and those who have been out for years, people who are displaced from their cultural base and people from *all* social classes, all use the team's services. It is time to throw out the stereotype of the 'vagrant alcoholic' and 'the skid row dosser', because they are the exception rather than the rule in the present homelessness milieu.

**The voluntary sector**

The second way of offering the team's service was through existing voluntary sector provision. St Botolph's Crypt Centre in Aldgate seemed an obvious choice on several counts:

a) The team had developed excellent links with the staff and clients there.

b) Drinkers were able to use the evening centre at St Botolph's as long as they did not drink on the premises.

c) The evening centre at St Botolph's regularly opened its doors to large numbers of single homeless clients.

d) Alcohol and alcohol problems had a high profile at the centre and the staff were interested in providing a service for this client group.

In addition, St Botolph's Day Centre had a 'dry policy' which meant it was able to follow up clients seen by the outreach team in a dry setting more conducive to positive work. There were also a whole range of health services available at the evening centre (provided by HHELP), including a general practitioner, a general nursing sister and a community psychiatric nurse, who, along with the centre's own social workers, could be usefully involved in a client's action plan.

Liaising with workers who were already providing a service at St Botolph's, it was decided that the team would offer an evening session on a Monday, for an initial period of six months to see what the uptake of the service was like. It was felt that Monday was a particularly useful time as it was the first evening session of the week and a time that many drinkers would have little money and might therefore be more inclined to use the team's services.

From the outset this service was regularly taken up by the clients of the centre. A great deal of joint work was undertaken and on over fifty occasions in a nine-month period the team were able to escort women and men directly to the Drink Crisis Centre. These clients were followed up by the resettlement team at St Botolph's. Again working together proved to be valuable to both clients and staff. Of those fifty clients, many have moved from the circuit to residential facilities such as 'Clouds House' in Wiltshire and others spent time away from the street, while their immediate health needs were taken care of. Contact has been maintained with almost all of them.

The outreach team from the Drink Crisis Centre was also able to work with an alcohol worker from St Botolph's to provide six 'alcohol awareness' training sessions for a group of centre workers. In these sessions, the stereotypes of alcohol and homelessness were challenged and workers asked to share their own attitudes about alcohol, in order to work more effectively with the client group. The team believe that working with people with alcohol problems is *not* a specialism, the skills needed to work with a person with alcohol problems are skills that all workers in the 'caring professions' should have at their disposal. What is needed is a transferring and enhancing of skills coupled with a knowledge of the service options available. This sharing of skills and knowledge is a vital part of the outreach team's work. The alcohol field has tended for too long to be a 'closed shop', excluding itself from the other caring professions to the ultimate detriment of the client group. The problems that alcohol produces are pervasive, affecting all social groups, and the more professionals able to provide a relevant service the better the chance of tackling the problem.

## THE WAY FORWARD

At the end of its first year of offering this service the outreach team has realized many of its initial aims. The team contacted a wide range of service providers in the fields of alcohol and homelessness and has worked with them in an attempt to provide a cohesive and integrated network of services.

It has offered, and continues to offer, a direct and regular service on the streets to women and men who are street homeless and are experiencing alcohol problems in their lives.

It has become a part of the street 'grapevine' and many people on the streets, certainly in Central London, are aware of the team's existence and the nature of the services offered.

The team have worked alongside existing outreach services, most notably the Rugby House Mobile Alcohol Team, Bondway Outreach, St Botolph's Crypt Resettlement Team and Thames Reach in an attempt to improve access to existing service provision.

It has referred and escorted over two hundred clients to a variety of service options, and as far as possible has stayed with them while they have been admitted or accepted into the service in an attempt to ease the transition from the street to the centre.

It continues to challenge and confront attitudes held by individuals and agencies about street homeless people with alcohol problems and has been involved in training and consultancy towards this end.

## WHAT NEXT?

Although all of the above sounds extremely positive there is a need to evaluate and to move on, and to realize that the team has done very little more at this stage than to improve the access to service provision for a small number of clients.

### Future goals

1 To work with the existing detoxification services in the voluntary and statutory sectors to render the service more accessible to the needs of women and men who are street homeless and in need of detoxification.
2 To look at the possibility of initiating a controlled community detox. within the existing voluntary sector, so that the single homeless person in need of detox. is not necessarily dependent on a residential service.
3 To refine the notion of a 'holding bed network' for individuals awaiting a detox. bed or a space in a recovery programme. This exists at the moment with Bondway and the Great Peter Street Hostel, but could be usefully extended, especially with the needs of single homeless women drinkers in mind.
4 To look at the needs of some of the different groups in the street homeless community, namely women, women and men from the

Scots and Irish communities, young people and those with mental health problems.

5 To continue to encourage and empower workers in the voluntary and statutory sectors to work with people who are homeless and have alcohol problems and to be able to refer them to relevant service provision.

What has been outlined in this chapter is a model of work. A model that hinges on respect for the client group, and a genuine commitment to improving access to service provision for the street homeless. It is a model that owes much to goodwill and to some good fortune, a model that hinges on co-ordination and co-operation, on putting aside one's own agenda and working together to achieve the best possible outcome. It is not new, it is not sophisticated, it is pragmatic, rather than academic, although it owes much to work that has been done before, most notably by Tim Cook at the end of the 1960s. If clients have found that they have been able to gain access to a service that they would not have felt able to use before, then it is a model which is both credible and has achieved a degree of success.

## ACKNOWLEDGEMENTS

To Rita Gannon who proposed that a crisis intervention model could be used at a 'street level' and Frank Moran who introduced the outreach team to the street community.

## REFERENCES

Cook, T. (1975) *Vagrant Alcoholics*, London: Routledge & Kegan Paul.
Heather, N. and Robertson, I. (1985) *Problem Drinking*, Harmondsworth, Middx: Penguin.
Procashka, J.O. and DiClemente, C.C. (1980) 'Towards a comprehensive model of change', in H. Heather and W.R. Miller (eds) *Treating Addictive Behaviours: Process of Change*, New York: Plenum Press.

# 6 Youth homelessness and health care

*Ian Boulton*

Britain has the fastest-growing youth homelessness problem in Europe.

(Shelter 1988)

Featuring in Shelter's 1988 report *A Place of My Own,* this observation came as no surprise to workers in the field. By the end of the 1980s it had become apparent to everyone, commuters, tourists, even policy makers, that the number of young people on the streets of the capital had reached epidemic proportions. The steady trickle of young working-class youth from the depressed industrial areas of Britain had become a flood. Until recently homelessness seemed to be confined to certain areas of the city, now the young homeless were everywhere; sleeping in doorways, begging on the street and in tube stations. The problem had become visible, could not be ignored and has not gone away.

While there has always been a street homelessness problem in Britain the recent upsurge in young homeless people sleeping on the streets makes them worthy of consideration as a separate category among the homeless population. This is true for a number of reasons.

First, the root cause of their homelessness may apply particularly to their age group. For example, it may be attributable to a breakdown in the local authority care system or to the introduction of a step-parent into the home. Second, the response of the statutory authorities, and the voluntary sector, will depend, to an alarming degree, on the person's age. Many voluntary agencies have a targeted age group of 16–21, believing that this group of homeless people have special needs which are best dealt with outside the wider homeless population. The statutory sector, in the form of local authority housing departments, will rarely place single people in their priority category, a system which discriminates against the young. Third, there has been a rash of legislation since 1985 which affects the lives of young homeless people directly. Some of these changes have led to the recent phenomenon of large-scale visible street homelessness among young people. Finally, there are specific health issues which are of greater concern to the young and those who work with them. AIDS/HIV and chaotic use of drugs may seem to be the most obvious of these, but this chapter aims to explore some of the other physical and mental health problems which face young people who have nowhere to live.

For these purposes we consider young homeless people to be those between the ages of 16 and 26 who are living on the streets, in occasional night-shelter accommodation or in temporary, disorganized squats.

For the most part they will also use some form of day-time facility, such as a day centre for homeless people, or be in touch with outreach or peripatetic provision. However, as well as the street homeless population, there are signs that young people under 25 make up over half of the hidden homeless population in London, i.e. those who do not present themselves to a recognized service. Obviously, there is not the same amount of information available about this group, but what little research has been done shows that, by concentrating simply on street homelessness, we ignore the scale of the problem among young women and those of black and ethnic origin.

The Threshold Project research into hidden homelessness in 1990 showed that over half of those surveyed were women, nearly two-thirds were under 25 and over half were of African, African-Caribbean or Asian origin. The main causes of their homelessness were overcrowding and family break-up. The effects of homelessness on the health of this group are similar to those who present themselves to medical services: stress, depression, weight loss, asthma, eczema and other nervous complaints. The paucity of services which attempt to meet the needs of young homeless women and young homeless people from the black and ethnic communities is in part due to the lack of information available about the hidden homeless population (Ye-Myint 1992). There is also a tendency to see street homelessness as somehow more serious. It would be more helpful if it was seen as the tip of the iceberg. By concentrating only on those people who have access to services, the apparent scale of the problem is diminished.

Within the 16 to 25 group there are also a number of subdivisions. While some of these divisions are of a somewhat arbitrary nature they are primarily the result of social legislation. For example, the 1988 Social Security Act which marked the end of general eligibility to benefits for 16- and 17-year-olds has had a major impact on the housing status of the under 18s. Second, voluntary agencies working with young homeless people use differing criteria in order to define their client group. Three West End agencies all within walking distance of each other variously limit their services to 16–21-year-olds (New Horizon), 16–25-year-olds (The London Connection) and the under 19s (Centrepoint). However, regardless of these arbitrary divisions this is an identifiable group with a common problem which can best be summed up as appropriate, accessible and affordable accommodation.

There is a remarkable consistency in the reasons individual young people give agencies for finding themselves homeless. Centrepoint report that nearly one-quarter of their clients have been through the local authority care system. Fourteen per cent, in 1988, had left home because of violence or harassment and there are significant indications that more young people are now identifying abuse as a prime or contributory factor to their homelessness. All the agencies interviewed, including Centrepoint and New Horizon, still maintained that half of the young people they work with left home to look for work. If this means they left home with 'unrealistic expectations' then they have been punished disproportionately for their mistake.

In 1985 the Conservative Government introduced board and lodging regulations which set a time limit for under 25s in bed and breakfast accommodation and rent ceilings which severely diminished the amount of temporary accommodation which was available to unemployed youth. This was the first of a number of major legislative changes which affected the lives of young people and contributed to the increase in street homelessness among the under 25s. As their options in terms of benefits, employment and accommodation were reduced, so many were forced to live outside the system.

1986 brought the Social Security Act, the abolition of supplementary benefit and the introduction of income support. The age-related benefits this entailed meant much lower rates for 16- and 17-year-olds and for 18- to 24-year-olds. This act also marked the end of single payments for deposits and rent in advance, replacing them with the Social Fund, an intractable system which causes delay and confusion at the very time when young people may see an end to their housing crisis. Under the 1986 Act, 19-year-olds in full-time education lost their right to benefits. Those still entitled to benefit now found themselves paid in arrears. If one accepts that low income remains the single most decisive factor in an individual's homelessness, then an act which deliberately sets out to make young people poorer must be deplored.

A further Social Security Act, in 1988, made youth training schemes compulsory for 16- and 17-year-olds if they were to receive any income. Within a few short months of this measure being introduced, a survey was carried out at New Horizon Youth Centre. They discovered that the average age of their client group had dropped from just over 20 to just over 18 between March and October of 1988. They also found that, whereas at the beginning of that year only 10 per cent of the young people using the Centre were sleeping rough, by November a staggering 80 per cent were on the streets or in squats. The same survey found a significant increase in the number of young women using the service, as well as a larger number of black youth and young people from the poorer boroughs of London. While the government promised a YTS placement to all 16- and 17-year-olds, no account was taken of the difficulty of keeping a job when you have got nowhere to live. The government also underestimated young people's distrust of these job training schemes. Many young people therefore learned from their older brothers and sisters that government training schemes, like Employment Training, were 'a con' and didn't help their employment prospects. So lots of 16- and 17-year-olds, far in excess of government estimates, simply decided to opt out.

The 1988 Housing Act hardly mentioned homeless people, never mind the young. The board and lodging regulations were removed in 1989, as were restrictions on people under 18 working in factories, mines and quarries and at night (1989 Employment Act). Furthermore, the 1989 Social Security Act stipulated that young people had to be actively seeking work in order to be entitled to claim benefit. These pieces of legislation collectively penalize young people by making them highly vulnerable to the risk of both homelessness and unemployment. Those young people faced with this prospect opt instead for low-wage, high-risk and often temporary work. Others are forced into working on a self-employed basis. When illness or personal difficulties occur, then many young people find themselves in the position of having their employment terminated and unable to claim full benefit for up to twenty-six weeks. It is not surprising that many of these victims of a punitive legislature find themselves out on the streets.

The causes of homelessness among young people not directly linked to government policy have more to do with the ways in which society treats its youth. These range from the role the young are expected to adopt within the traditional nuclear family to the treatment of those brought up in the care of a local authority.

In most nuclear family structures, there is an expectation that the children will be able to support themselves financially upon completion of their education. In periods of high unemployment these expectations cannot be fulfilled, placing an intolerable strain upon relationships in poor families. The situation is sometimes further aggravated by a transition, for example the introduction of a step-parent or the break-up of the marital home. Indeed, it is these often traumatic events that have been identified by workers in the field as a major cause of youth homelessness. Some young people find themselves being ejected from the family home either because they have had one argument too many or simply because the family can no longer afford to feed them. They may also feel guilty because they can no longer pay their way. A number of agencies have reported that the chronic rise in youth homelessness over the last decade has mirrored the unemployment patterns of the period. In 1981, Central London agencies working with young people identified their client group as coming from outside London, from Glasgow, the North East, Liverpool, Belfast, South Wales, the depressed industrial areas of Britain. Poverty had driven them from their homes to the prosperous South East. By 1988, young people from the poorer boroughs of London made up 50 per cent of New Horizon's clients. Centrepoint and Soho Project and the other Central London agencies were finding the same.

As well as being a time for starting work, of course, the end of education is also meant to mark the time when young people are free to live independently. Late adolescence is represented in our culture as a time of financial independence, a time to experiment and have fun before 'settling down'. Whilst this has never been a reality for working-class youth, young people do feel a tremendous pressure to live up to the role and the role models presented to them. The attraction of London for the young, disaffected and disenfranchised is probably a result of these pressures.

And if living up to the role expected of you is difficult for those brought up within a family, what of those whose parent is the State? Many homeless young people have been brought up in local authority care and there are a number of reasons why the care system has contributed to the homelessness statistics.

For example:

1 Inadequate preparation for independent living. Many young people

leave the care system without even the most basic knowledge of the benefit system or of skills such as budgeting or how to cook a simple meal.

2 Lack of support systems. While every young person has the right to support from local authority social services, in an era of cost limiting and service cuts they form just one of many competing demands on the system.

3 The care system often fosters an over-reliance on others and a belief that those 'in authority' will come to the rescue. Survival skills learnt in care equip young people to live in groups rather than independently.

4 Many young people find the instability of some local authority homes too difficult to cope with and leave the system and either return home to an equally unstable home situation or simply run away. In doing so they often lose contact with those whose responsibility it is to place them in independent accommodation.

A comparatively small percentage of people who have grown up in families leave home on their eighteenth birthday to live alone. For most people the experience of leaving home is gradual, with many returns to the family home, before they become fully independent. They have the chance to experiment, to make mistakes, to be bailed out by the family and friends now and then.

Young people who have grown up in care are not allowed to make mistakes. Failure to manage money and pay the rent regularly results in eviction. The local authority, far from behaving like a 'good parent', shows little sympathy towards those it has been responsible for once they are technically adults. Therefore it is hardly surprising that young people from care form a large percentage of the young homeless.

From the moment a young person enters the care system, whether they are 6 months, 6 years or 16 years, careful thought should be given to their future. Drifting through a succession of children's homes and foster placements without a clear plan for the future does not help children develop the sense of identity and confidence they will need to survive after the cut-off point of their eighteenth birthday when professional support is usually abruptly withdrawn.

It is almost unnecessary to make the point that, although many young people have chronologically reached adulthood, they have the emotional needs of much younger children. Yet these 'children' are expected to live alone, hold down full-time jobs or be in full-time education, manage a tight budget and be sensible way beyond their years. Some of them have children of their own. Some of them have been placed in private and voluntary establishments in rural areas throughout their childhood, but must return to inner cities to be housed.

It is possible to understand the preference many young people show for street life, with its myriad and transitory friendships, over the isolation and boredom of a bedsit or flat in a tower block.

Those who leave the care system early by running away have, in the past, forfeited their right to housing. There are many reasons why young people run away from care but the predominant factor is that their placement is not acceptable to them. Involving young people in the plans made for them is essential if this problem is to be tackled.

Other young people simply outgrow care and want to experience life on their own terms. If, however, they make this decision when they are 17 they find themselves in the position of being too old to be received back into care and too young to be independently housed.

Finally, there are a disproportionate number of black children within the care system. It follows that this group will become over-represented among the homeless.

The Children Act of 1990 placed a duty on local authorities to accommodate 16- and 17-year-olds 'whose welfare is likely to be seriously prejudiced'. CHAR, the campaign for housing rights say in their report on the act:

> Local Authority Housing departments in liaison with Social Service departments need urgently to plan provision for young people under the Act:
>
> – levels of accommodation provision for young people will need to be increased;
> – Housing Associations and voluntary agencies will need increased financial support to extend their provision of housing for young people in need;
> – efforts will be required to explore and respond to the needs of homeless young people more effectively.

The report also emphasizes that more information and evidence about young people is needed if the opportunities provided by the Act, particularly in relation to accommodation, are to be grasped.

The link between abuse in the family home and homelessness is a cause of increasing concern for workers in both the voluntary and statutory sectors who come into contact with young homeless people. They are finding that more and more young people are prepared to talk about this issue as either the root cause or a major contributory factor to their housing crisis. An experienced youth worker at New Horizon comments:

> It would have been almost unthinkable when I first began here that a young man or women would talk about abuse at home in the day centre. It would have been far too dangerous for them. You know, what if they don't believe me? What if I'm the only one? But now it's quite common for that to happen which is sad, but encouraging that they feel they can speak out. Obviously, we are not a specialist facility and it's not necessarily an appropriate place for those with complex emotional needs to attend. But where else can they go?

A large percentage of homeless young people are now revealing that they ran away from home because they had been sexually abused. In some cases they run to escape an abusive situation. Others run because their abuse was undetected or because they felt blamed for what has happened to them. The effects of sexual abuse in childhood can be seen in adolescents who 'act out' their feelings of worthlessness by running away and becoming involved in drug abuse and prostitution. Many under-age prostitutes, both male and female, reveal that they were sexually abused as children.

The choices open to these young people are frightening. They can stay at home and continue to be abused or run away to a risky, uncertain lifestyle. The third option, to speak out to the authorities, is often not even considered because the taboos against breaking up family life, combined with irresponsible media coverage of sexual abuse cases, act as a deterrent. Unfortunately, some young people run away because they have been abused while in local authority care, so fear the authorities which are meant to protect them.

Any attempt made by a young person to escape an abusive situation should be seen as a courageous act. Agencies need to support such actions by providing shelter and counselling to runaways. Training in these matters for workers in the voluntary sector is essential. There is also a desperate shortage of 'safe houses' for these young people. The responsibility for such provision needs to be accepted by all local authorities.

Just as young people are vulnerable to becoming homeless, they are also vulnerable to ill-health. This is the product of a number of different but interrelated factors.

Young people with nowhere to live are often overwhelmed by the difficulty of just surviving. Such difficulties are made more extreme when the young person develops even a minor illness. Coughs, colds and other influenza-type illnesses are both more prevalent and at the same time likely to take longer to shake off. Being young and homeless the sufferer cannot simply change their lifestyle. There is no recourse to bed, a warm environment or a nourishing meal.

Similarly, cuts, burns and all manner of abrasions take longer to heal when the young person is living in a squalid and unhygienic environment. Thus dressings become filthy and sodden, providing a perfect medium for bacterial infection, or fall off altogether.

Young people wearing ill-fitting or inappropriate footwear are often found to have badly excoriated feet leading in some cases to hospitalization. Numbers have risen in recent years with the increasing popularity among young people of training shoes. These are often worn for days at a time as the owner dare not risk removing them either for fear of theft or because they are aware that their feet have become so swollen that once off they will not be able to put their shoes or trainers back on.

The homeless existence also leaves many young people vulnerable to mugging or other forms of physical attack. This is not an uncommon phenomenon and often results in the victim being released from a casualty department as if they had somewhere to recuperate. 'Off the Streets', a project for young people based in Dean Street, cite the example of a young person who had been hit over the head with an iron bar who spent three days in a shop doorway trying to recover.

Young people are also in some jeopardy when faced with the problem of taking prescribed drugs. This may be because they don't possess a watch and so have little or no idea how long has elapsed since their last pill or because their medication is stolen or lost. The example of asthma is sometimes cited by workers in the field. This is not an uncommon condition, one which the majority of housed sufferers manage to cope with extremely well. For those out on the street it is a different story. They find that, when they come to use their inhalers, they have gone astray or they haven't managed to register with a GP and so don't have a repeat prescription.

Many homeless young people, particularly those who are new to the streets, are extremely poorly prepared for the demands that homelessness makes of them. Unlike their housed peers they have generally made an extremely abrupt transition to independence and are inadequately prepared for the alien world of homelessness. Young people in this position need rapidly to develop a set of basic survival skills such as a sense of distrust and a knowledge of the network of day centre and hostel provision. While some are adept at developing such informational and coping mechanisms, many do not. Such young people are in a position of maximum risk. Amongst the most vulnerable are those who have left home because their parents can no longer cope with their behaviour. Many such 'difficult' teenagers are displaying the early symptoms of mental disorder such as schizophrenia, leaving home feeling traumatized, confused and depressed and come to medical attention only after a serious crisis has occurred. Other young people with mental health problems have been discharged from mental hospitals and have for one reason or another lost contact with those whose responsibility it was to provide them with help and support.

Particularly vulnerable are those who become homeless as a consequence of sexual abuse. These young people may become entrapped into the equally dangerous and destructive world of prostitution. Entrapped not in the sense that they are lured into prostitution by pimps waiting to ensnare them at mainline railway stations, but because for so many prostitution is a continuation of a vicious circle of self-loathing and contempt. Emotionally damaged and often without any formal qualifications, young people enter prostitution because it may seem to be the only means of supporting themselves. For some it may also be the only means they have of exercising personal power and controlling their environment. Either way, prostitution is not a positive choice but an occupation which is associated with poverty, despair and risk.

Even young people who are highly aware of the risks of unprotected sex and have an in-depth knowledge of HIV and AIDS may be unable to act upon it. Some young people lack any sense of personal power and so do not feel able to resist demands for unprotected sex. Others may be so emotionally damaged that they don't care.

Such young people may also use drugs regularly or be experimenting with them in the same w ys as many of their housed counterparts. However, unlike the latter, many homeless young people find that they are less able to take the necessary precautions in purchasing and using drugs in order to ensure maximum safety. Indeed, evidence suggests that drug use among homeless people tends to be more chaotic, a case of using whatever is available or affordable without knowing exactly what they are taking let alone the side effects. This may entail glue sniffing because it induces a cheap effect or injecting the dissolved contents of prescribed drugs such as Temazepam. This practice can result in the amputation of a limb as the dissolved jelly which is melted prior to injection can solidify, leading to thrombosis formation and occlusion of the blood supply to arms and legs.

Those who do want to curtail their drug usage face the almost impossible task of waiting for a hospital bed to become available in order to detoxify, as few drug rehabilitation centres will take addicts who are not drug free. This is a major undertaking for housed drug users let alone homeless ones. Indeed, many find themselves caught in a vicious circle as there are few hostels willing to admit drug users and provide them with the support they require. Faced with the choice of withdrawing while living on the street or in a squat or continuing their drug use it is unsurprising that the majority choose the latter.

This highlights one of many major gaps in provision which affect the young homeless and even exacerbate their situation. Few young people know how to register with general practitioners and therefore use accident and emergency departments when they are sick. This is problematic for a number of reasons: first, because, unlike a GP, the accident and emergency department does not have access to the young person's medical record. They may also not be aware that the person they are treating is homeless. This lack of knowledge concerning the individual's medical history and housing situation can lead to danger-ous practice. 'Off the Streets' cite the example of a young homeless girl who suffered from epilepsy and had been taken off her anti-epileptic drugs after a visit to out-patients and sent away with an appointment to see a neurologist in three weeks. The problem was that without medication the girl was suffering from frequent fits which in the context of being on the streets was extremely hazardous.

While some agencies provide specialist medical provision for the homeless many of the people working in the field of young homeless people see this as a dangerous precedent. Many feel that rather than marginalizing the homeless by segregating them from mainstream provision the health care system should be adopting a more flexible response. This might mean, for instance, not discharging the sick on to the street but allowing them to convalesce in hospital. As a worker at the New Horizon day centre argued, 'Homeless people need more care from the Health Service, not less.'

A recurring theme when talking to those whose work brings them into contact with the young and homeless is 'safety'. The word crops up again and again in conversation. It appears in day centres' and night-shelters' stated aims and objectives, in annual reports and funding applications ('We aim to provide a safe and comfortable environment where young people can . . .'). It was also the word most often used when a group of young people were asked what they thought should be done to ease the youth homelessness problem.

– There should be a safe place for people to go to recover from illness

or injury. For the housed population, this would be the convalescence period spent at home. Either hospitals need to reassess
their policy in relation to homeless people, allowing them to stay in
until they are fully fit, or never discharging someone onto the
streets, or special sick-bays should be set up to meet this need.

- Local authority safe houses are needed so that abuse in the home
  does not lead to homelessness.
- Young people experiencing mental health crises need access to
  short-stay crisis intervention facilities, similar to those which exist
  for drug users.

The young women and men who came up with these solutions clearly
see the rise in youth homelessness as a symptom of society's failure to
protect its young. The response to the crisis has been dispiriting:
piecemeal, with a ludicrous over-emphasis on Central London and
little or no preventive work in the rest of the country. There has also
been an over-reliance on small-scale voluntary services which will
never be able to cope with the problem nationally. These services have
become vital and should be supported. Whilst voluntary agencies are
bearing the brunt of the youth homelessness crisis they should be
assured of their continued existence. It is not acceptable that the vast
majority of these agencies are forced to stumble from one financial
crisis to the next. Their funding must be secure.

There must also be adequate training offered to workers in voluntary sector agencies. A worker in a day centre is expected to know how
to deal with a wide range of difficult problems and situations. Too
often, they are thrown in the deep end without training or support.
This results in a high staff turnover and a poor service for clients.

In the end, however, only a far-reaching strategy which places the
emphasis on statutory responsibility for our young people can help to
eradicate homelessness among the under 25s. Fundamentally, all
homeless young people should be accepted as vulnerable under the
1988 Housing Act. Only then would the government be going some
way to ensuring that future generations of young people are not faced
with having to make choices about their future out of desperation.
This already occurs in some London boroughs which accept 16- and
17-year-olds as vulnerable. A youth support service, based within each
local authority in the country, is also needed. This would provide a
more holistic approach to young people's issues, offering welfare
rights, counselling and access to a range of services covering areas like
leaving home, the care system, abuse, mental health, education and

employment. Only a society which offers this sort of support has the right to be surprised when something goes wrong.

## BIBLIOGRAPHY

NAYPIC (undated) *Abuse in the Care System*, National Association of Young People in Care.
NAYPIC (undated) *Report on the Violations of the Basic Human Rights of Young People in Care*, NAYPIC.
Newman, C. (1989) *Young Runaways*, London: The Children's Society.
Thornton, R. (1990) *The New Homeless*, London: SHAC.
Ye-Myint, C. (1992) *Who's Hiding?*, London: NFA.
Young Homeless Group (1990) *Unsecured Futures*, second edition, YHG.

# 7 Models of health care provision

*Elizabeth Bayliss*

Both primary and secondary health services often find it difficult to be sufficiently flexible to meet the varying needs of their users. This inflexibility affects people who are home-based as well as homeless and many of the issues raised in this discussion will have relevance for other people besides London people whose circumstances preclude them from easily fitting into the established systems of health care delivery. For instance, people who are illiterate or whose mother tongue is not English might well find it difficult to access the services they require.

It is to be hoped that the changes we are now undergoing within the Health Service, the Family Health Services Authority and the social services will provide us with the opportunity to adopt a more flexible approach, based more on a functional response to the actual individual needs of users, dictated less by stereotypic presumptions and implicit judgements of personal worth.

Various initiatives have been taken to secure health care for homeless people. Some have aimed to provide direct physical care in environments familiar to homeless people; others have aimed to intercede with the health services to secure access to standard services, on behalf of homeless people. All start from a recognition that homeless people on the whole are not well served by our statutory health services.

How best to provide health care for homeless people is the subject of lively debate. It centres on a judgement as to whether it is better to accept the fact that the Health Service cannot be changed and concentrate on the here and now, treating as many individuals as possible, directly, in an environment separated from the rest of the population, or whether it is better to put effort into trying to make the Health Service adapt to meet the actual needs of all homeless people, referring them into mainstream services for treatment on an integrated basis.

Using this axis, three models of health care provision for homeless people can be characterized as follows:

Separate services
Special schemes that assess and intercede
Fully integrated services.

Each of these models will be viewed from four angles: access, care, environment and coverage, as laid out in the SHIL Report.[1]

## Access

I shall be asking whether services are easily available when required; who has access and on what terms; whether the services are well advertised in places homeless people find themselves and whether the primary services can organize access to secondary services, when required.

## Care

What range of treatment is offered by the services provided – do they include dental, ophthalmic, psychiatric, chiropodial, as well as general medical; is the standard of care offered adequate; does the treatment offered promote positive health, as well as treating illness?

## Environment

Do the services continue the segregation of homeless people; do they assist homeless people into decent housing or confirm them in their dispossession; do they assist in changing the immediate environment of homeless people?

## Coverage

Who is reached by the services provided? We should remember the diverse nature of the homeless population and take into account that women who are homeless may have some different health needs from homeless men; black people and people from different ethnic communities again may have different requirements. The health profile of young people will not look like the health profile of elderly people who are homeless. In addition, people who are living on the streets are likely to present with physical complaints that differ from those of people living in large hostels.

## SEPARATE SERVICES

### Ethos

The inspiration for the development of separate services exclusively for homeless people comes from a recognition that standard services are never likely either to give priority to homeless people nor to respond appropriately to their needs. It is considered unrealistic, and a diversionary waste of energy, to attempt to bring about change. More to the point is the provision of direct treatment for some people at least. Advocates of separate services sometimes suggest that homeless people prefer separate services because separation means that they are not subject to the prejudices of home-based people. It is considered kinder to segregate not just to protect against a hostile world but also to allow homeless people to feel comfortable in a familiar environment. Thus, separate health services are traditionally provided in hostels or day centres or walk-in clinics that cater exclusively for homeless people.

Up and down the country, new proposals for walk-in clinics for homeless people are regularly being developed as a response to the seemingly hopeless task of persuading the mainstream services to provide enhanced access.

For example, the Bridge Project in Newcastle[2] is a walk-in clinic for homeless people. Southwark Day Centre in South London[3] has developed a proposal for a separate service and in acknowledgement of the failure to secure access to health, the King's Cross Project,[4] which provides support to homeless people including families and single people, is aiming to establish a separate walk-in service.

### Access

Access is easy for residents of the traditional hostels, resettlement units and day centres served by their own medical staff. With the service provided on site there is no need even to go to a drop-in medical unit. In walk-in clinics too, for those that know about them, there is a high level of acceptance of all who come, with no receptionist restricting entry and no appointment needed. Such separate services may provide a means of access to secondary health care but this might well take the form of a sick-bay, when what is really needed is the full range of medical back-up only available in a hospital.

## Care

In hostels and common lodging houses where separate services are often poorly funded, they usually consist of nursing services which co-ordinate the health input, backed by a visiting medical officer (VMO) employed to visit the establishment for a certain number of hours each week. In many cases, other separate services are gradually added, such as dentistry, chiropody and sick-bays. Southwark Day Centre's proposal for a walk-in clinic includes a sessional GP or nurse practitioner and a health worker providing direct care.

Within the sort of 'total environment' provided by traditional hostels, however, the workers' personal knowledge of their clients can form the basis of real preventive care, over a period of time. People can be treated more holistically, though expectations may become fixed in such a containing regime, with the consequence that residents might find it difficult to change.

Despite their limitations separate services often do have the capacity to operate with real flexibility, capable of listening to individual clients drawing on a range of skills innovatively. It is within separate services that the potential of the controversial role of nurse practitioner has been explored most fully. For example, the activities of Barbara Burke-Masters in East London generated the energy that led to the creation of HHELP.[5]

## Environment

Nevertheless, the forces of institutionalization are strong and, within the closed environments of traditional hostels, such forces are likely to embrace both carers and clients. It is easy to stay within the safe confines of the building and its fixed relationships. Carers and clients might both have low expectations of the clients' ability to move on to independent living. Expectations of positive health may be lower because of environmental conditions reducing the chances of real health. Absorption within the institution may reduce the motivation to challenge inadequacies in mainstream services.

Walk-in clinics are not likely to be so self-absorbed, though inherent in the provision of separate services of any kind is the danger that workers will become marginalized alongside their clients. Change in mainstream services becomes inconceivable; challenging services a waste of valuable effort. This attitude gives rise to the litany: 'There is no point in raising people's expectations by having them register on the housing waiting list because they will never be given priority for housing and there is no point in pressing the local GPs to provide a responsive service for our clients because they will not be accepted for fear of frightening away other patients who will not want to associate with them, even if only in a waiting room. All we can do is ensure that homeless people are as comfortable as possible.' Over time such assumptions can become ingrained, passed on from one generation of workers to the next. Staff then find it difficult to draw on wider community resources and provider networks. Separate services might protect clients but at the long-term cost of perpetuated segregation.

## Coverage

Separate services tend to cater only for people who have been homeless for a long time, who use traditional facilities for 'the homeless'. This represents a very limited response. No attempt at comprehensive coverage is usually made, even within the homeless population. The problem here is that there are many people who are disadvantaged who do not identify themselves as homeless as such and who would not see their interests as coinciding with those of 'the homeless'. For instance, if a homeless person is a young, black woman, it is unlikely that she will identify with a service that caters predominantly for middle-aged white homeless men. The danger is that other health providers might well assume that the separate service is indeed comprehensive and appropriate for all homeless people. The young black woman might then find herself, effectively, denied access to any health service at all.

## Comments

The advantages of exclusive services are plain to see: ease of access for those who know about the service and the ability to focus the delivery of care to a very specific group of people. However, it is often the case that local general practitioners will feel relieved of all responsibility to accept a homeless person onto their lists because of the existence of such a separate service. People who are homeless are channelled through segregated provision, whether they identify with that provision or not.

The danger with separate services is that they risk helping in the containment of homeless people, confirming their segregation away from the rest of society. The long-term interests of their users would be better served if they functioned less to offer direct treatment and concentrated more on advocacy work: doing assessments of need, establishing working links with the local primary and secondary health and social care services, working with local health promotion units and establishing referral rights to the local housing agencies.

There are some pockets of good practice in operation, where workers are indeed engaged in bridging the gaps between segregated, institutional provision and mainstream health and housing services. For example, the clinical nurse specialist at West London Day Centre[6] sees her role as building therapeutic relationships with homeless people who do not often expect to be healthy and assessing individual people's health, housing and income maintenance needs. She provides continuity of care so that, when a client comes back from hospital, she tries to make sure they are fully informed about their after care. She works on treatment and care plans, integrating housing needs into these.

She does not always succeed in fulfilling her role to her own satisfaction. For instance, when it comes to providing continuity of care, this can prove extremely difficult when she is not allowed access to the doctor's notes or not told what treatment one of her clients has been receiving while in hospital.

In conclusion, separate services tend to cater only for certain groups of homeless people, doing little to help people escape from the subculture of homelessness.

## SPECIAL SCHEMES TO ASSIST HOMELESS PEOPLE

### Ethos

The motivation for the establishment of special schemes is the recognition that the health services are biased against homeless people and that this is not acceptable. Homeless people should be informed of their rights and help should be available to enable them to secure these rights. Both general practice and hospitals should be encouraged to provide services without discrimination. Active intercession is required to achieve this aim. Special schemes focus on assessing people's needs and advocating on their behalf for access to mainstream provision. Such schemes tend to see people as a whole and provide advocacy and support in relation to health, housing, resettlement and benefit needs. Thus, they tend to be multidisciplinary teams.

I shall be looking in some detail at two special schemes, both set up by the Department of Health in 1986 as three-year pilot projects with a remit to assess the morbidity of and provide open access health care to single homeless people in London. Both have developed their work quite considerably over the past seven years. The East London Homeless Health Project (HHELP) initially consisted of a salaried GP, a community psychiatric nurse, an alcohol worker, a nursing sister, a social worker and a co-ordinator. Primary Care for Homeless People (PCHP),[7] the second of the DoH-funded pilots, originally consisted of a nurse, a locum GP and administrator. Currently, PCHP has two nurses, a health advocate, fifteen sessions (two hours each) per week undertaken by local GPs and a GP facilitator, who does two sessions per week.

At the end of the three-year pilot period, following a major appraisal of the project's progress, and in accordance with the objective of encouraging their clients into mainstream primary health care, the salaried GP in the East London team was replaced by nine local GPs working with the team on a sessional basis. At the same time, the Department of Health direct funding of the pilot was replaced by a combined package of long-term secure funding from the local statutory authorities that has resulted in the team becoming a permanent part of local health care provision. The team now comprises a manager, the sessional GPs, administrators, social worker, resettlement worker, CPN, a nursing sister and an alcohol worker. Recently, further DoH funding has been secured for a three-year period to develop an outreach service for homeless people with mental health problems. This brings another CPN, social worker and resettlement worker plus two generic outreach workers and a psychologist into the team.

**Access**

Access is seen as a key issue. Opening up access to mainstream health and other services is a prime function, though not the only one.

GP surgeries and group sessions are held by HHELP in local day centres and hostels which cater for homeless people, so access to the services of the team is limited. Consequently, although access to mainstream services is a prime purpose of the team, the contact point with homeless people is within segregated settings.

Likewise, the places in which the GPs do sessions for PCHP are places for homeless people, such as day centres and hostels. One interesting development though has been the establishment of a weekly session for women who are homeless, held in Elizabeth Garrett Anderson Hospital.

## Care

Special schemes consciously aim to act as a bridge, sitting between separation and integration. They have a dual objective: gaining access to general services on an integrated basis, on the one hand, and providing direct transitional primary health and social care services on the other.

The HHELP team offers, through surgeries and groups, primary health care, counselling, social work and resettlement services. Once resettled, their clients are registered with a local GP and receive services on an integrated basis. One problem the team encounters is the lack of continuity in the GP service: it is difficult to make coherent a care programme for individuals which may involve several GPs. It is through the sessional GPs, however, that referrals to the team are made. Their involvement in the team is thus vital and a networked computerized medical record minimizes confusion.

The team resolves the tension between assisting with access and providing a direct separate service by emphasizing the fact that the clinicians in the team are employees of the mainstream services: District NHS Trust, Family Health Services Authority or local authority. The line managers of team members sit on the management committee of HHELP. Problems of access are brought to the managers who are expected to work them out within their authorities.

PCHP defines its role as identifying clients' needs and providing care where there is no other provision. It aims to facilitate access to mainstream services. With other service providers, PCHP engages in training about homelessness and health. The two nurse specialists act as practitioners and provide continuity of care. The health advocate works with other providers to assist homeless people in need of health services who are referred by the local authority housing department homeless persons unit.

## Environment

The HHELP team considers its strength to lie in its multi-agency, multi-professional nature, enabling it to respond to the interrelated problems of clients in a way which enhances their opportunities for reintegration.

A striking feature of the cohort of people seen by PCHP is the fact that all the clients have complex problems, only one of which is their health. The conclusion reached by the PCHP staff is that a multi-professional approach is vital. They find it essential to work closely with other agencies since so many clients have other problems beside ill-health.

## Coverage

HHELP saw 2,500 clients between 1987 and September 1990; fifty new clients are seen each month, with one hundred consultations a week. Coverage is not comprehensive since the services are accessible only to those people who use the homelessness agencies where HHELP runs its surgeries and groups. Women are particularly under-represented.

A greater attention to outreach within HHELP is expected to result in contact being made with a broader range of people on the streets, who are not currently in contact with any other service.

PCHP operates in Camden and Islington in London, where in Camden alone there are estimated to be 5,000 homeless people. In 1990, 625 people were seen by PCHP, half of whom were sleeping out. Sixty-eight per cent of the people had had no medical contact at all in the last six months.

## Comment

It is perhaps interesting to note that both teams see themselves as having an advocacy role, although it is only PCHP that has formalized this role into a specific job. Advocacy is an important new concept within the health and social care arena, in which professionals (or volunteers in some settings) take on the job of speaking up on a person's behalf. It is a good example of the way that services for homeless people have had to be innovative in order to promote their clients' welfare in a relatively hostile environment. Useful lessons, transferable to other health care services can be learnt from such client-centred ways of working. Practical solutions that purposely blur the distinction between health and social care can indicate the way forward for mainstream services.

Another example is the post of salaried GP. Although this post has now been dropped from the HHELP team, in order to encourage a broader responsibility through using local GP practices, the idea of creating a salaried GP post to provide primary health care to a targeted group of people has not been lost. Much of the initial work in the formation of a relevant contract is likely to prove useful in a wider arena and has already been taken up in Leeds where the Health Care for Homeless People Project[8] has a salaried GP. Out of hours GP back-up is provided by a co-operatively run health centre.

## FULLY INTEGRATED SERVICES

### Ethos

At the other end of the spectrum from separate services are fully integrated services. The problem here, though, is not only one of access to existing health services. The problem is the organizational ethos of our National Health Service. It is rigid and leads us to feel that we must fit in or risk not receiving a service at all.

Its rigidity requires the would-be user to follow procedures and operate a flexibility more appropriate to the provider than the recipient. It is for this reason that, implicit in seeking integrated services, is a demand for change. Separate and special schemes offer the Health Service lessons on the way forward.

### Access

For homeless people to secure access to primary health care, they have to be able to register with a GP. Where an active attempt has been made to increase registration, considerable success has been achieved,[9] if expectations are clarified on all sides. Homeless people may need encouragement to register and GPs may seek assistance before agreeing to accept patients. Other patients of the GP may need to be reassured.

Homeless people though are often accepted only as temporary rather than permanent patients. The supposed mobility of homeless people is the usual justification. However, a Department of Environment national survey found that 63 per cent of homeless single people had lived more that one year in their current county, while more than 40 per cent had lived more than a year in their current district or borough.[10]

The problems of access to health care vary according to the circumstances of the homeless person. If a homeless person is living in a large hostel, common lodging house or resettlement unit, the task of securing registration with a local GP could be hindered by the GP's anxiety about being swamped by demand from the hostel, which might 'upset' their home-based patients. If a homeless person is living in temporary accommodation, such as a bed and breakfast hotel, they might not wish to register with a GP local to the hotel. They might feel that to do so would be to sever yet one more vital link with the area identified as home, thus heightening the sense of rootlessness. The task here would be to ensure temporary registration. If a homeless person is living on the streets, they may need to have their entry assisted. The initial task here would be to make contact with the homeless person. Workers would make contact with individuals directly on the street, as do the HHELP outreach team.

Information on services available should be disseminated locally and conspicuously advertised in the form of posters on street hoardings, near bus stops and DSS benefit offices. They should describe how to gain access to health care in the case of homelessness. They should be visible in all local languages.

### Environment

The under-resourcing of primary health care was recognized by Harding in 1980[11] and the demand to give greater priority to the provision of primary care and relate it to local needs and secondary health services has been growing steadily since then. Compounding this pressure to increase the capacity of primary care is the development of community care and the local reprovision in place of long-stay hospitals, which by definition inevitably places more responsibility on primary care providers for people previously cared for by secondary providers.

The creation of budget-holding GP practices, where GPs are able to buy whatever specialist services they think most appropriate for their patients within the constraints of their practice budget, gives us a glimpse of the real issues at stake in shifting the power balance between primary and secondary health care. GP fund holders are not tied to purchasing only services on offer from their local district health authorities or trusts. They can purchase from wherever the relevant specialist service is. It has made health authorities pay attention to the views of their 'home' GPs. The many inequities occurring in the present GP budget-holding system should not cloud the potency of this attitudinal change.

The formal division between the purchasing and providing functions as defined in the National Health Service and Community Care

Act 1990 has further provided an opportunity for the local community and GPs to comment on health authority priorities. Secondary health providers are now required to work to contracts, whereby the volume, quality and type of their provision is specified and performance is monitored by the purchasers. Although it is easy to become confused by the ideology of the NHS internal market, the most important concept of contract specification opens up the debate about health service priorities, giving local purchasers the opportunity to look at performance and to target priorities for action, which has not really been possible before. The needs of homeless people could be built into the contract specification process. Public health departments are usually advising local purchasers on priorities, on the basis of their local analyses of need, so it is these departments which must be persuaded to undertake research into the needs of homeless people in their area.

**Care**

Lack of good management and organizational coherence in health services frequently confounds attempts at a flexible response. Currently GPs are independent contractors who can employ their own staff, while community nurses, such as health visitors and district nurses, are employees of the district health authority or trust. The two different systems of management and organization do not aid an integrated and co-ordinated approach. The Cumberlege Report[12] recommended the establishment of primary health care teams based on formal agreements describing the aims, objectives and roles of the participant doctors and nurses, however employed.

Some real change in the profile of health care could emerge from the pilot work being done in Yorkshire and other places where family health services authorities and regional health authorities are exploring how to develop a coherent management structure and thus allow genuine multi-professional primary health care teams to develop, involving GPs, community nurses, health visitors, occupational therapists, community psychiatric nurses, physiotherapists, etc. It would be even better if these teams were not made up solely of health workers but included housing and social workers as well.

It is increasingly widely recognized that change in working relationships between primary and secondary health care providers is essential. Currently, communication is often very poor, with a hospital stay regarded as an 'event' unrelated to the patient's life before or after admission. The Medical Campaign Project found in their research into health care needs of single homeless people that two-thirds of those interviewed had left hospital without discussing with staff where they would go on discharge.[13]

The Medical Campaign Project for improved access to health care for single homeless people[14] recommend a seven-point action plan for adoption by hospitals on discharging homeless people. It specifically looked at the needs of people coming out of mental health units, but its eminent sense makes many of the points useful for application to all areas of health care. The action plan covers ward staff training, the provision of a community psychiatric nursing service to hostels and day centres used by homeless people, an out of hours service, liaison with magistrates' courts, access to convalescence beds and production of an information booklet.

From April 1991, health authorities have been statutorily required to introduce a care programming approach for patients with long-term mental illness. The intention is to ensure that patients treated in the community receive the health and social care they need by:

i) introducing more systematic arrangements for deciding whether a patient referred to the specialist services can, in the light of available resources, the views of the patient and his/her carers, realistically be treated in the community.

ii) ensuring proper arrangements are then made, for the continuing health and social care of those patients who can be treated in the community.

(DoH 1990: 80)

Any mechanism that helps build bridges between hospitals and their local communities should be sincerely welcomed. What is unfortunate, however, is the context within which this initiative sits. Many hospitals are having to cope with real demoralization: many inner-city district health authorities are having to reduce their level of activity in order to stay within budgets that are too small. The sense of despair is often held at bay by a sharp resentment to yet more change, yet more requirements. Whilst government directives can be interpreted as cynical gestures, full of words and empty of resources, effective implementation will not follow. Indeed, when the future seems so uncertain, holding onto what we already have, however inadequate, can be represented as an achievement.

If our National Health Service survives, with a continued commitment to the provision of services free at the point of delivery to everyone in need and with a strengthened primary health care sector, care planning could give us a solid bridge. The directive that hospitals agree local arrangements for implementation with their local authority social services and the requirement that hospitals work with their non-medical colleagues in co-ordinating both a patient's health and social care needs are most welcome. It is only through inter-professional working that a really responsive, client-centred service can be assured. The pity is that the legislation does not extend to cover everyone in priority need with long-term ill-health. For homeless people, in particular, such an approach could prove useful.

Within a multi-professional framework, using an individualized care plan, primary and secondary health care providers could co-ordinate their work with informal carers and other professionals. The circumstances of a person who is homeless would become evident and remedial action would be identified with the responsibility for action allocated. If a person had a chronic health problem, or ongoing support need, responsibility for ensuring appropriate support would be allocated to a key worker. The success of such a model depends upon the flexibility of the providers and their willingness to see the person as a whole. For instance, a key worker trained as a community psychiatric nurse might have to spend an inordinate amount of time helping their client secure the full DSS benefits to which they are entitled when they move into their flat. Or because their client is keen to meet other elderly people from the Caribbean, they might spend time finding out the address of a local lunch club for Caribbean elders. This sort of activity might be considered more of a priority than booking an appointment to see the doctor! It is unfortunate that such a concept of flexibility is so often interpreted ideologically as a mechanism to bring care costs down by de-skilling professional workers. Start from the point of view of the service user in that debate and the effect of such professional flexibility can result in the empowerment of the user and their carers.

Real integration demands not only flexibility but regular liaison and the development of active networks among service providers in a local area, many of which are likely to be voluntary sector agencies. For homeless people in particular, the development of active, co-ordinated networks among health, housing, income and social support agencies would represent a real improvement in service provision. An attitude of partnership should be fostered, with the voluntary sector given a place in the local joint planning process alongside statutory agencies, carers, advocates and users themselves, in recognition of the increasingly strategic role voluntary agencies are planning.

## Coverage

Homeless people are often invisible to service providers. The only visible homeless people may well be those who seem to correspond to the stereotype. In a recent study undertaken in East London to establish an impression of the number of 'rough sleepers' or people living on the streets with nowhere else to go, 1,100 people were identified, over half of whom were refugees.[15] Local demographic profiles and analyses of need often omit mention of homeless people. With the introduction of community care plans, it has become even more important for homeless people to be counted in the local description of need, since central government funding to local authorities will flow according to an as yet unknown formula related directly to defined local needs.

Compounding this anxiety, health authorities will in future receive their funding from the government on a capitation basis, assuming a certain level of need per head of the population. Some weighting for poor areas is likely, to take account of the increased health needs of the population in areas of high deprivation, which should include the needs of at least a part of the homeless population. If their needs are not counted properly it will result in an insufficient financial base. What is already certain is that increased resources are urgently needed if we are to allocate resources to the members of our society whom we have so far failed.

In inner-city areas, where homelessness is increasingly such a visible issue, public health departments and purchasers are advised to establish health development (homelessness) posts with the dual brief of establishing the real extent of homelessness in an area and identifying ways in which needs could be met within the local pattern of services. In the process of drawing up the local map of homelessness, post holders would raise local awareness about the scale of the problem, pressing for an integrated local response from different health authorities, family health services authorities, local authority social services and housing departments, voluntary organizations, housing associations, service users and community groups. It is in the joint consultative committee that these different bodies decide on matters of joint interest where agreement should be sought about local priorities for resource allocation.

## CONCLUSION

Separate services and special schemes are both responses to the failure of the Health Service to provide properly for homeless people. Full integration for homeless people may be the ideal but only in a more flexible and responsive health service and most practitioners consider the obstacles to achieving this insurmountable. If they are right, special schemes provide the most constructive and pragmatic way to proceed, working as they do to bring about change in the Health Service slowly and with specific relevance to the needs of individual people.

The separation of purchaser and provider functions does give an opportunity to bring about some lasting changes within mainstream services that could result in a better health service that responds to the needs of homeless people. The contracting process opens up for debate decision making about priorities. If these were determined locally according to the identified needs of the population health gains could be measured by looking at the health of the local population. The absorption of the Health Service with its own service systems would thus be shifted into a more relevant client-centred context. Factors such as the potential power of the GPs *vis-à-vis* hospital-based consultants, an emphasis on care planning for individuals with long-term health and social needs, the growing significance of community care and the development of advocacy suggest the opportunity for long-term improvements.

It is the extent to which their practitioners aim directly to bring about change in mainstream services that characterizes the difference between the three models of health care provision for homeless people that have been discussed in this chapter.

Separate services give priority to the provision of a direct medical service to a specific group of homeless people in a segregated setting. Access into mainstream services is seen as an unrealizable ideal that diverts energy away from dealing with the immediate health needs of some homeless people.

Special schemes, too, try to respond to the primary health care needs of their clients but on a transitional basis, placing equal emphasis on advocating to achieve access to the range of services needed by their homeless clients: primary and secondary health care, support, social care, housing, help with resettlement. They provide the model for integrated services, outreaching to homeless people from a multidisciplinary team base while retaining contact with their mainstream colleagues and employers. The limitation of special schemes lies in their rootedness in segregated settings for homeless people which means their coverage is partial and limited to people who categorize themselves as homeless.

Integrated services go further along the same path as special schemes in creating access to mainstream services. The difference between the two really lies in the target population. Special schemes have so far tended to target a particular section of the homeless population. Integrated provision starts from an assumption that comprehensive coverage is the goal and that service provision should reach out to meet unmet needs in whichever way is necessary to ensure an effective response. From this broader base, it should be possible to find ways to reach more people without a home base, such as people who are refugees.

It is evident now that it is precisely by targeting services to meet the particular needs of a specific group of people that the NHS can respond effectively. It is the establishment of a whole range of special schemes, advocating on behalf of different particular groups, that will create the flexible service demanded on condition that such special schemes operate in a multidisciplinary way embracing social care in seeking a positive and holistic response.

Consequently, to build on the success of the special schemes, a series of outreach teams, providing primary health and social care specifically for homeless people would be developed. Keeping the principle of integration in mind, such teams would operate on a locality basis, co-terminous with the other locality-based primary care services in an area. They would aim to provide a comprehensive service to all homeless people in their area, providing direct care and advocating on behalf of their clients with mainstream health, housing and social providers.

It is essential with such special schemes to avoid marginalization, in order to prevent them becoming outposts, with no route back into mainstream services. This can be avoided by the establishment of posts within the authorities' central planning and contract management networks to promote the interests of particular groups of people with specific needs. For example, the appointment of health liaison workers in family health services authorities would be supporting special schemes by working with GPs to create a pool of doctors with whom homeless people are welcome to register. Building this vital first link with mainstream services through GPs would then not be left to the workers on the ground. Liaison workers could undertake training of DHA and FHSA clinicians about homelessness, thus easing the pressure on the voluntary agencies and front-line workers in securing access. They would work with training departments to raise awareness of the health implications of economic realities and social deprivation, challenging the clinical categorization of homelessness which diminishes the seriousness and complexity of the issues involved.

With respect to strategic planning and co-ordinated care delivery, health development workers (homelessness) would focus on increasing recognition of the extent of homelessness in the local area. They would ensure that homeless people's health, housing and social needs were quantified by public health departments and that co-ordinated services were planned and budgeted for in provider contracts and community care plans.

In conclusion, such changes do not represent a radical break with current practice. Special schemes are already showing the way. Their experience provides a good base on which to build the wider networks of connections that would ensure more comprehensive coverage. Given the severity of the problems faced by homeless people and given the increasing government expectation that agreement should be reached locally about priorities, it becomes urgent that the needs of homeless people are formally recognized and that they are given priority. Indeed, an understanding that positive models of integrated health and social care for homeless people can guide provision for all groups with special needs should give us the necessary impetus.

## NOTES

1 Bayliss, E. and Logan, P. (1987) *Primary Health Care for Homeless Single People in London: A Strategic Approach*, SHIL (Single Homeless in London) Health Sub-Group.
2 The Bridge Medical Centre, The Close, Quayside, Newcastle upon Tyne; telephone: 091-241 7189.
3 Southwark Day Centre, 81 Camberwell Church Street, SE5 8RB; telephone: 071-703 8877.
4 King's Cross Project, Gregory House, 48 Mecklenburgh Square, WC1; telephone: 071-833 3775.
5 East London Homeless Health Primary Care Team (HHELP), 42 Carnegie House, 20 Osborn Street, London E1 6TD; telephone: 071-247 7232.
6 West London Day Centre, 36 Seymour Place, London W1; telephone: 071-402 5468.
7 Primary Care for Homeless People (PCHP), 92 Chalton Street, NW1 1HJ; telephone: 071-387 1241.
8 Health Care Team, FHSA, Brunswick Court, Bridge Street, Leeds LS2; telephone: 0532 450271.

9 Bayliss and Logan, op cit., pp. 20-4.
10 Department of the Environment (1981) *Single and Homeless*, London: HMSO.
11 *The Primary Health Care Team*, report of a Joint Working Group of the Standing Medical Advisory Committee and the Standing Nursing and Midwifery Advisory Committee, chaired by Dr Wilfred Harding, 1981.
12 Department of Health and Social Security (1986) *Neighbourhood Nursing – A Focus for Care*, report of the Community Nursing Review, chaired by Ms Julia Cumberlege, London: HMSO.
13 Medical Campaign Project (MCP) (1990) *Good Practices on Discharge*, The Print House, 18 Ashwin Street, London E8 3DL; telephone: 071-249 2560.
14 Medical Campaign Project, op. cit.
15 No Fixed Abode (NFA) (1991) *Rough Sleepers*, 2nd Floor, The Brady Centre, 192-6 Hanbury Street, E1 5HJ; telephone: 071-247 0285.

# 8 Research or campaigning?

Raising the profile of health care for single homeless people

*David James*

Concern for the housing needs and welfare of the homeless is not a recent phenomenon. In 1890 General Booth published *In Darkest England* where, among many recommendations for the improvement of services to the poor, he called for clean lodgings and model suburban villages. He argued that 'one of the first steps which must invariably be taken in the reformation of this class, is to make for them decent, healthy pleasant homes . . .'. To emphasize the necessity of decent housing Booth referred to the homeless of Trafalgar Square where, in the latter part of the nineteenth century, large numbers of homeless men camped out as they had nowhere else to shelter. As a first step towards improving health care of the homeless poor, Booth recommended using a pony and trap together with two nurses to dispense basic health care. An early example perhaps of outreach work?

General Booth's reports and speeches had a dual purpose: to mitigate the miseries of the poor and homeless and to propagate the gospel. While his extravagant language and Christian zeal may seem misplaced today he set an agenda that would not basically change throughout this century. Campaigns after Booth would be tied to a succession of research projects that attempted to discover the true situation of the poorest in society.

After General Booth with his message of social selection and salvation came the two great social researchers Charles Booth and Seebohm Rowntree with their categories of the deserving and non-deserving poor. These definitions would blight social reform throughout the following century. However, their research undermined the view that poverty was an expression of personal choice and demonstrated that its main cause was social circumstances such as old age, low pay or lack of employment.

How much these findings and the campaigns that sprang from them influenced the Liberal Government of 1906 and its social reform programme is debatable. The impact of the Boer War and the fear of physical inadequacy within the population resulted in the creation of a Committee on Physical Deterioration in 1903. It reported little evidence of deterioration but did state that working-class health and nutrition left a great deal to be desired. Added to this was the fear of declining 'National Efficiency'. The Liberal Government was also aware of the growing strength of the labour movement in terms of both trade unions and the fast emerging Labour Party. These factors were probably stronger influences upon the policy makers of the day than any research into poverty. However, the campaigning of Booth and Rowntree probably contributed to a change in attitude towards the poor by some powerful and influential groups in society.

Research by both Rowntree and Charles Booth attacked the entrenched stereotypes of poverty. Their findings demonstrated that poverty affected a wide variety of people, from the elderly to young men working for inadequate wages. Similarly, homeless people are stereotyped as drunken old men, but in reality anyone, given certain circumstances, could find themselves without adequate shelter. In *Down and Out in Paris and London* published in 1933 George Orwell described his fellow travellers as being:

> of all kinds and ages, the youngest a fresh-faced boy of sixteen, the oldest a doubled up, toothless mummy of seventy-five. Some were hardened tramps, recognised by their sticks and billies and dust darkened faces; some were factory hands out of work, some agricultural labourers, one a clerk in a collar and tie, two certainly imbeciles.

> (Orwell 1933)

Whatever their background, homeless single people and the very poor prior to World War II could not and did not expect easy access to health services. However, with the establishment of the National Health Service and its commitment to equality of access free at the point of delivery, politicians could claim that the UK had a comprehensive health service that served the needs of all the community. From these fine beginnings came disillusion and reassessment with the findings in the 1980s by, first, Professor Black and later Anne Whitehead that the Health Service did not treat the community equally. Rather, as the health demands of the most vulnerable grew, due to poverty and poor housing, the actual service they received declined proportionally. The 'Inverse Care Law' first defined by Tudor Hart was reinforced and reached its zenith with the homeless whose access to health services was restricted and often actively discouraged.

While the housing and health care needs of single homeless people have, until recently, been ignored, research into the 'causes of homelessness' has prospered. In 1975 at a meeting held under the auspices of the DHSS, which concerned itself with the needs of single homeless people, David Brandon talked of a 'buoyant gloom' in research into homelessness.

According to Brandon, there were mountains of research papers but still 'Himalayan' heights of homelessness. The authorities were more than willing to fund research but they seemed unable or unwilling to act upon its findings. This situation was compounded by the fact that researchers felt themselves limited by academic orthodoxy and, therefore, shied away from making radical proposals, fearing ridicule from practitioners in the field or from other researchers. Papers were often magnificent in diagnosis but lukewarm when it came to making recommendations. Furthermore, taking on the role of secular priests, researchers seemed incapable of talking in a language accessible to practitioner and layperson alike. This meant only a select few could understand and interpret their findings.

This pessimistic view of the capacity of research to act as a catalyst was dominant in the late 1970s and early 1980s. Workers in the field, together with umbrella organizations and campaigning groups, achieved a modicum of success by highlighting the inadequate treatment and care of the single homeless by health care providers. CHAR and the Association of Community Health Councils used the following example to campaign for a more adequate and receptive treatment of single homeless people in accident and emergency departments.

Mr X was taken by two Brighton housing trust workers from where he was sleeping to the accident and emergency department at around midnight. He was sleeping rough on Brighton beach. He had substantial rectal bleeding, for which he was undergoing treatment from a sympathetic GP. He was in considerable pain and suffering and our GP was not prepared to set a precedent by going on to the beach to treat people, so we had no choice. On arrival at casualty he was seen by a receptionist and details were taken – he was told a few minutes later that it was not an emergency and he should go and see his GP.

(CHAR/ACHCEW 1980: 5)

A local campaign was set up to ensure that this situation would not occur again. Various levels of management within the local health care service were contacted. The subsequent debate led to a commitment from the local hospital to give full access to treatment; referral, during the day-time, to a local day centre for onward referral to a GP or, at night, ensuring that the person was fit to leave the hospital and giving them a list of GPs who would see them next day, together with a copy of their medical notes from casualty to assist the GP in giving speedy treatment; and finally a commitment given to run educational sessions for medical staff.

A similar situation which gave rise to a national debate concerned Thomas Frazer at Hackney Hospital. In August 1978 Mr Frazer, a 57-year-old homeless man, fell down in the street and was taken by ambulance to Hackney Hospital and examined by the casualty officer who was never told he had fallen heavily. The doctor pronounced him drunk. Frazer was told to leave the hospital but only did so when the police were called to get him to leave. Then he walked out by himself, outside he fell down again and was brought back into the hospital by some ambulance men. The casualty officer did not know that Frazer had left and had been readmitted and did not re-examine him, so the diagnosis of drunkenness remained. The police were again called, but they refused to charge him with drunkenness and take him into custody. He fell down again in casualty but little attention was paid to him. He was then taken to a police van and transported to the local station. There no one knew what to do with him and, after some debate, he was taken to a local churchyard and left on a bench. He died a few hours later of a brain haemorrhage caused by a fractured skull.

This tragic event led to an investigation by the City and Hackney Community Health Council who produced a report entitled *Homeless and Healthless* (Fowke *et al.* 1980), which found that the local health services failed to provide adequate health care to the homeless.

After the report was published the issue was raised in the House of Commons by Ernie Roberts, MP for Hackney North and Stoke Newington (*Hansard* Vol. 989, No. 224, Col. 1475). He cited the Hackney CHC findings, which recommended that homeless people should be encouraged to register with local GPs and that GPs be persuaded to accept them on their lists. The need to educate medical staff concerning the reality of homelessness was emphasized, something achieved locally in the Brighton area after the case of Mr X. The link with the GP service, argued Mr Roberts, was essential so that single homeless people could access mainstream services, as they should be able to as of right.

Mr Roberts received a reply from the then Under Secretary of State for Health and Social Security, Sir George Younger (*Hansard* Vol. 989, No. 224, Col. 1480), who demolished the idea of separate services for the homeless. Instead, he strongly supported the idea that single homeless people should register with a local GP, although he recognized the difficulties some homeless people might encounter. The government clearly saw registration as the means of delivering health care to homeless people.

Mass registration by single homeless people was not, and did not become, a reality. In 1984 Barbara Burke-Masters, nursing sister at the St George's Mission on Cable Street, London was still shocked at the poor medical care or advice received by the homeless. She made contacts with local GPs and hospital consultants, but in 1985 her efforts were stopped by legal action initiated by the pharmaceutical society. However, her actions and concern led to two relevant outcomes: first, a great deal of publicity was generated which embarrassed the statutory authorities into action; second, the actions of Burke-Masters helped raise the expectations of the homeless themselves who reacted well to her formal and thorough service. But easy access to the mainstream was still problematic.

In 1986, some six years after the debate between Ernie Roberts and Sir George Younger, the Medical Campaign Project was established as a result of the difficulties residents of the Simon Community had experienced when attempting to gain access to medical treatment. The project had three main aims: to campaign on behalf of homeless single people for improved access to existing health services; to educate health professionals about the needs of homeless people; to increase publicity about these issues in all areas of the media: a familiar list to those working with the homeless but a condemnation of the lack of progress achieved in gaining access to mainstream medical services during the first half of the 1980s.

The campaign for improved medical services holds within it a tension, in the conflicting objectives of pursuing a service for the 'here and now' or attempting to convince the authorities and vested interests that only access to the mainstream can guarantee comprehensive health care services. Throughout the 1980s three possible strategies have been debated: separate services, special schemes and mainstream services. These were summarized by Elizabeth Bayliss in the previous chapter.

Mainstream service, the preferred means of health care delivery, is one that has been most avidly campaigned around by agencies in the field. However, GP services as presently constructed would not be able to cope effectively with the needs of homeless people within the community. GP services are often locked into the need for registration and, in most cases, operating rigid appointment systems that cannot respond to the requirements of homeless people who need a more flexible approach. An essential prerequisite would be education of health care providers in order that stereotypical conceptions of single homeless could be challenged.

This strategy brings into question the basic structure of the GP service as it suggests that a multidisciplinary approach would be beneficial not only to single homeless people but also to the wider community. This would reflect a general shift of resources away from the hospital sector and towards the community.

By integrating homeless people into mainstream services, the stigma of their situation would be diluted and hopefully eradicated. A multi-disciplinary approach would involve closer liaison with local authority services such as housing and social services and the accident and emergency units to prevent individuals being discharged without support.

As the 1980s progressed it became increasingly evident that single homeless people were encountering substantive difficulties in accessing health care. While campaigning organizations frequently attempted to engage the interest of policy makers they failed to attract either the funding for new developments or policy changes.

In *Health Care for Single Homeless People* (Williams and Allen 1989); it was reported that two-thirds of professionals and representatives of voluntary groups felt that single homeless people needed special and separate provision of primary health care services. However, this was for many a short term expedient with integration being the long term aim. Clearly they had not heard of the J.M. Keynes maxim 'in the long term we are all dead'.

The very establishment of separate services takes the pressure off mainstream providers to develop the flexibility to cope with the needs of single homeless people.

For instance, in *From the Margins to the Mainstream* (Stern *et al.* 1989), the authors make a powerful case for integration while at the same time recommending the development of a separate walk in clinic primarily for the use of homeless people in the proximity of Waterloo Station. It has been argued elsewhere that special services, if they are to be operated, should be within the confines of a local accident and emergency department.

SHIL have also criticized the concept of special schemes. 'The value of such special services relies upon being able to make a long term impact on the thinking of the regular providers of services, not only the health service but also in the voluntary sector and the statutory, local authority services. They will not do so by being outside. This is where the homeless find themselves' (SHIL 1987). SHIL also went on to point out that in social policy terms such schemes are rootless as they are not linked to a framework for policy planning and as a result are often marginalized.

The PSI report also points to the shortcomings of specialist services. In summarizing the activities of a number of specialist schemes, the authors, Williams and Allen, pointed out that, while the services these offered were of a high standard, there were certain drawbacks. The care offered was available only on certain days and the schemes were often channelled through day centres, night-shelters and hostels. A whole section of the homeless population was not reached because its members did not use those services. Also, some individuals already registered with a GP used the project GP as an alternative source of medical treatment.

The authors also cast doubt on the necessity for multidisciplinary teams. They pointed out that there were problems with team management and, as they were separate from mainstream provision, the team structure actually got in the way of providing an effective service.

A major critique of short-term schemes is that their long-term aim of increasing registration with local GPs is often not achieved and the PSI report supported this view. Clients felt they were receiving mixed messages from the GP who treated them but at the same time suggested they go elsewhere. Clearly this would not be the situation if the service being offered was strongly rooted within the mainstream health service.

The PSI felt that special schemes had offered a good service, often in difficult circumstances, but they should not be seen as the answer to the problem. In fact, the very existence of a distinct and separate service continued the marginalization of single homeless people. The belief of the authors was that mainstream provision should be made more flexible so as to meet the primary health needs of the majority of the single homeless. Multidisciplinary elements of team work needed to be included in any mainstream provision and then targeted at those homeless individuals who have specific health needs.

Education has always been seen as an important method of increasing medical staff's awareness. This is all very well and the authors of the PSI and numerous other reports mention it with tedious regularity but, without financial inducements, little progress could be expected or achieved. This does not simply mean the payment of doctors but also the supplying of resources that allow for the recruitment of extra ancillary staff to support the provision of a wide-ranging primary care service. This would have the benefit of helping all those in the community and not just the homeless, so reducing the stigma often carried by the group.

The 1980s started with the recognition of the poor health service on offer to those people who are defined as homeless. Questions were asked in the House of Commons, albeit at 1 am, and awareness of the issue was undoubtedly raised. Numerous groups have reported and campaigned throughout the period, especially as the number of homeless began to rise. The response of the government has been negligible and the housing crisis continues to deepen, with the lack of affordable council housing plus rising repossessions in the private sector making homelessness a problem that will continue into the 'caring 1990s'. So what has changed? The issue of health care provision to the homeless population has often been seen in terms of short-term projects and research-based initiatives. Only at Christmas does the charity 'Crisis' succeed in obtaining major media coverage of their efforts to supply food, shelter and care for the homeless over the 'festive season'.

In relation to the long-term development of policy and a campaigning strategy, the Medical Campaign Project, which began as a short-term endeavour, continues to work and develop awareness into the 1990s. It is probably a reflection of the lack of success during the 1980s in convincing the government to resource health provision that in the early 1990s the Medical Campaign Project continues to exist.

As a fundamental principle MCP makes the important point that the NHS, based on equity and access, fails to deliver a service to the homeless in the community. In the 'final report' of 1988 the Project reported large gaps in medical provision; where provision did exist, only white males were catered for, raising the important issue of the hidden homeless. This hidden element would include groups such as ethnic minorities and women, the latter being found less often on the streets or in hostels though they may well bed down with friends while having no home of their own.

MCP have documented the difficulties faced by single homeless people in attempting to register and hence have called on voluntary sector organizations to recognize health care as being as important as welfare or housing rights. It is apparent that the issue of health has not been properly addressed by the campaigning charities who operate in the area of homelessness.

Interestingly, one of MCP's original aims was to 'increase publicity about these issues (homelessness and health) in all areas of the media'. Yet in the 'final report' (1988) it was noted, in connection with a conference held and organized by MCP in June 1986, that only local media covered it, but this was not seen as a negative factor. It was felt that the raising of awareness among service providers was more important. This perhaps reflects the limited time and resources available to inform relevant media outlets, but also the *internal* nature of the debate concerning health care for the homeless. The education and training of professionals within the health and voluntary sectors is often given greater priority by campaigning groups. There is a belief that change can be achieved through internal pressure rather than external pressure through public concern.

MCP's campaigning efforts, as with most groups linked to homelessness, have been, and still are, narrowly focused. This involves lobbying of Members of Parliament from all parties and persuading members to ask direct questions to relevant ministers. This has often led to answers that illuminated the government's lack of understanding of all the issues in relation to homelessness. MCP have highlighted questions put by Charles Irving in 1987, which led to a government response that suggested that the right to access medical care together with two special projects in Tower Hamlets and Camden District was all that was required to guarantee access. Health authorities and family practitioner committees were also targeted to discover how they were approaching the issue of health and the single homeless. In 1988 only West Lambeth DHA, as mentioned earlier, had a working party but generally London DHAs had not addressed the issue. FPCs' responses were patchy and, although some like Kensington and Chelsea had looked at the issue of homeless families, generally little across the capital had been done.

It is important to understand that MCP, as the only organization that campaigns exclusively on issues of health linked to the single homeless, limits its activities to London. It is noticeable that the vast majority of research into homelessness and particularly health issues has a London bias.

MCP has also taken on a training role, which links well with a campaigning approach that places the influencing of professionals above informing the general public. Professional bodies such as the Royal College of General Practitioners and the Royal College of Nursing were targeted. Contact was made and in the case of the Royal College of General Practitioners a seminar was organized for deans of faculties, regional advisers, FPC administrators and representatives from the DHSS. It was hoped that raising the issue of health care and single homelessness with the medical profession itself would lead to changes in the training of future GPs. The Royal College of Nursing also agreed to take part in a similar seminar jointly planned with the

CHAR National Health Group. Whether or not the seminars had the desired effect is debatable but there is no doubt that the issues have been successfully highlighted, if not acted upon.

At the end of the 1988 'final report' the Project could conclude that 'The DHSS has no real overview and, while some DHA's and FPC's are reviewing local need, none to date have clear, implemented policies' (MCP 1988).

The Royal College of Nursing/CHAR conference restated what had been said in the 'final report' of 1988, that the Department of Health had no comprehensive policy in relation to single homelessness. It pointed out the problem of communication that existed between individual voluntary organizations and statutory organizations such as DHAs. This issue remains a major problem affecting the effectiveness of campaigning in the area of homelessness, as different philosophies and structures are often a barrier to communication.

The conference highlighted the complex issues and problems faced by homeless people and those who attempt to campaign on their behalf, an interesting area which may develop into the campaigning thrust of the 1990s is the reaffirmation that homelessness affects distinct groups such as ethnic minorities, the mentally ill, the elderly and women.

The need to build coalitions between single homeless people, campaigners and established interest groups is evident. Homeless people are in a weak position to assert their rights, not least because they are effectively disenfranchised by their addresslessness. Therefore, if partnerships can be formed and information exchanged, organizations with resources and structure, like Age Concern or MIND, could be utilized. The growing awareness that groups such as the elderly are suffering homelessness and, therefore, greater ill health is an opportunity to place the issue on the government agenda and inform the general public. CHAR have also emphasized the importance of coalition building in areas of common concern. They recommended that joint working should take place with organizations such as MIND and patient activist groups.

The development of coalitions would lead to the formation of a much stronger campaigning platform which would have a more powerful voice, one that might raise public awareness and influence professional behaviour.

While both research and campaigning have heightened the profile of issues surrounding health care and homelessness, what has led to the greatest change in attitudes has been the greater visibility of homeless people on the streets of our major cities. Demands for action have been heard from many quarters, but to a large extent the voice of homeless people has been silent. Images of homelessness, often conforming to the mythological stereotype, have 'spoken' on their behalf, leading to misconceptions and inappropriate responses. It is essential that campaigning organizations and coalitions empower homeless people by calling on their experience in order to legitimize their actions and to speak with an authentic voice.

## BIBLIOGRAPHY

ACHCEW/CHAR (1981) *Health and the Homeless*, London: ACHCEW/CHAR.

Andrews, K. and Jacobs, J. (1990) *Punishing the Poor*, London: Macmillan.

Booth, W. (1890) *In Darkest England*, London: Salvation Army.

Central London Outreach Team (1984) *Sleeping Out in Central London*, London: GLC.

CHAR (1989) *Health Care for Homeless People*, London: CHAR.

CHAR (undated) *Single Homeless People and the Health Services*, London: CHAR.

CHAR/ACHCEW (1980) *Primary Medical Care Provision for the Single Homeless: Findings of ACHCEW survey*, London: ACHCEW/CHAR.

Cook, T. (1979) *Vagrancy; Some New Perspectives*, London: Academic Press.

DHSS (1975) *Report on the Proceedings of Meeting Held on 13/3/75 to Discuss Research into the Needs of Homeless Single People*, London: DHSS.

Fowke, B., Turner, T. and Coulter, P. (1980) *Homeless and Healthless*, London: City and Hackney Community Health Council.

*General Practitioner* (1987) 'Expect some harsh words from Sister Barbara', June.

*Hansard* (1980) *Parliamentary Debates*, Volumes 989 and 224, London: Hansard.

Hay, J.R. (1975) *The Origins of Liberal Welfare Reforms 1906–1914*, London: Macmillan.

Hirst, L. (1988) *High Care Housing*, London: SHIL/SITRA.

Leach, J. and Wing, J. (1980) *Helping Destitute Men*, London: Tavistock.

Medical Campaign Project (1988) *Final Report*, London: MCP.

Medical Campaign Project (1990) *A Paper Outlining Good Practice on Discharge of Single Homeless People with Particular Reference to Mental Health Units*, London: MCP.

Medical Campaign Project (1991) *Healthcare and Single Homelessness: A Conference Report*, London: MCP.

O'Connor, P. (1963) *Britain in the Sixties: Vagrancy, Ethos and Actuality*, London: Penguin.

O'Neill, M. (undated) *Resettlement Units: A Review of the Literature*, London: DHSS.

SHIL (1986) *Single Homelessness in London*, London: SHIL.

SHIL (1987) *Primary Health Care for Homeless Single People in London: A Strategic Approach*, London: SHIL.

SHIL (1988) *Single Homelessness among Black and Other Ethnic Groups*, London: SHIL.

Stern, R. *et al.* (1989) *From the Margins to the Mainstream*, London: West Lambeth HA.

Thane, P. (1982) *The Foundations of the Welfare State*, London: Longman.

Whaley, K. *et al.* (1989) *The Future of Primary Health Care for the Single Homeless in East London*, London: City and East London FPC.

Williams, S. and Allen, S. (1989) A *Summary of Health Care for Single Homeless People*, London: PSI.

Wood, S.M. (1979) 'The social conditions of destitution: the situation of men with schizophrenia', *Journal of Social Policy* 8 (2): 207-37.

# 9  The American experience

*Jim Reuler*

During the decade of the 1980s, homelessness in the United States evolved from being a backwater problem confined to isolated pockets in larger urban areas to a major societal issue impacting on most geographic areas in the country. Recognition of this growing problem was highlighted by the fifty-five-city survey of hunger and homelessness published by the U.S. Conference of Mayors in late 1982, which was followed soon thereafter by the first hearings on homelessness in the U.S. Congress since the Great Depression.

Since that time, the societal, legislative and media attention focused on homelessness has emphasized the harmful effects on health caused by lack of shelter. Homelessness can be considered as a reversible environmental state which places a growing portion of the poor in the United States at high health risk. Homelessness makes people sick.

The plight of the homeless epitomizes the relationship between politics, social policy and health. The absence of national right-to-housing laws and lack of any semblance of an organized health care system in the United States are both problems which extend far beyond the purview of health professionals. However, the myriad adverse health consequences of homelessness have become very much the concern of the health professions. Recently, professional societies such as the American Medical Association, the American Public Health Association and the American Academy of Pediatrics have published position papers from symposia held to focus attention on this problem and to develop strategies for improving the plight of this most disadvantaged group of the medically needy in the country. As well, the health consequences of homelessness have become an area for academic study. In addition to numerous journal articles, four major texts on health care for the homeless and the findings of the National Academy of Science's Institute of Medicine study on health care and homelessness have been published. This chapter will provide an overview of homeless care and recent initiatives in the United States for improving health services delivery to this group.

## DEMOGRAPHICS OF THE HOMELESS

The size of the homeless population in the United States remains a topic of much debate (Wright 1989). Estimates in the mid-1980s by the Department of Housing and Urban Development placed the number of homeless at around 300,000 nationally, whereas homeless advocacy groups, extrapolating from local surveys, placed the number at closer to 3,000,000 individuals. Marked discrepancies in these figures reflect different definitions of homelessness, methodologic issues of the surveys and the political persuasion of the reporting agency. More recent authoritative opinions place the number of homeless individuals in the United States on any given night at 800,000. At the beginning of the 1990s, it is estimated that 3–4,000,000 individuals are homeless in the United States over a one-year period of time. In large urban areas such as Los Angeles, as many as 33,000 individuals may be homeless. For the first time, the United States census, conducted every ten years, has included a special effort to count the number of homeless in the country. Forthcoming information from the 1990 census may provide more accurate accounting of homelessness.

The Institute of Medicine survey defined a homeless person as 'one who lacks a fixed, permanent, night time residence or whose night time residence is a temporary shelter, welfare hostel, transitional housing for the mentally ill or any public or private place not designated as sleeping accommodation for humans' (Institute of Medicine 1988). A number of factors have contributed to the increasing numbers of people who meet this definition, the most important being the decreasing availability of low-income housing in the country. Between 1970 and 1980, 50 per cent of the single room occupancy (SRO) hotel units available in urban areas across the country were lost to demolition or gentrification. During this same period, the aggregate supply of low-income housing decreased by an additional 2.5 million units, while federal support for subsidized housing decreased over 60 per cent. The decreasing availability of low-income housing coupled with the increasing numbers of people living in poverty have forced many people into a state of perpetual homelessness. Decreasing government support for publicly financed cash benefit programmes has frayed further this tenuous safety net for the poor. With increasing unemployment, fewer benefits available and rising housing costs in urban areas, many individuals and families must choose between shelter and other basic necessities (Linn and Gelberg 1989; Wood *et al.* 1990).

One of the most striking aspects of homelessness has been the changing demography of the population. Whereas previous analyses of homelessness in the United States identified a homogeneous group of older, white alcoholic men who were poorly educated, recent studies show that there has been a dramatic increase in the heterogeneity of the homeless population. Figures published by the U.S. Conference of Mayors in 1987 show that only 56 per cent of the homeless population was comprised of single men, whereas 25 per cent were women and homeless families represented 28 per cent of the total, the majority of this group being children under the age of 5 (Bassuk and Rosenburg 1988). The median age of the homeless population in the United States is now 34 years, and only 20 per cent represent the typical 'Skid Row' population of earlier years. Also, one-third of the homeless population is comprised of veterans of military service, many of whom are chronically impaired due to their experiences in the Vietnam conflict and estranged from social support and health care services.

The chronically mentally ill account for about 30 per cent of the homeless population and are a vulnerable group for whom health care delivery is particularly problematic (Lamb 1984). In 1955, there were 559,000 patients in state mental hospitals across the country. The community mental health movement, civil rights advocacy and the development of effective psychopharmacology fostered the concept of deinstitutionalization and the development of programmes to shift care of the mentally ill into the community. As a result, the population of state mental hospitals had fallen to 132,000 by 1984. Unfortunately, implementation of the community-based component of this deinstitutionalization programme has not been realized, with only a fraction of projected community mental health centres funded. The inadequate community mental health support and the economic hardships many chronically mentally ill face have resulted in an enlarging population of disaffiliated mentally ill individuals who are homeless on the streets of many urban areas and who cycle through the criminal justice system because of the behaviour consequent on inadequately managed major mental illness.

The decreasing age of the homeless population, the increasing numbers of women and children within this group and the disproportionate representation of minority groups and the mentally ill have changed the character of the homeless population and have broadened the issues facing health delivery planners (Bachrach 1987; Weinreb and Bassuk 1990).

## HEALTH CARE DELIVERY IN THE U.S.

Whereas a primary tenet of the National Health Service in Great Britain is to provide comprehensive care to all, a right to health care has never been established in the United States. That no system for health care for the homeless exists in the United States is not a surprise considering the fact that the United States is the only major industrialized country without a national health programme. In a nation abundantly endowed with hospitals, doctors and advanced health care technology, millions of citizens have difficulty obtaining health care, and the homeless are the most disenfranchised of this group (Robertson and Cousineau 1986).

Health care for the homeless must be viewed in the context of this non-system of care and the mechanisms for health care financing. As there is no universal health care programme for all citizens, access to health care for most people is determined by the level of an individual's insurance coverage. Private health insurance is available to many Americans through their place of work. Over 1,500 private insurance companies offer coverage in the United States, with many differences extant regarding benefits covered, exclusions and costs. Unfortunately, many small businesses cannot afford to provide health care insurance as an employee benefit, accounting for the fact that two-thirds of uninsured Americans, some of them homeless, live in families with at least one full-time employed worker.

Two major public health insurance programmes arose out of the Great Society legislation of the mid-1960s (Fein 1986), based on the idea that investment in 'human capital' would create a more cohesive and productive society. Medicare (Public Law 89–97; Title XVIII of the Social Security Act) covers the elderly over age 65 and certain categories of the disabled. This programme uses public dollars to pay for services delivered by, and in, the private sector and is governed by a single set of rules which apply nationwide. Medicare covers only 44 per cent of the medical expenses of the elderly, requires out-of-pocket deductible and co-insurance payments by beneficiaries and, since it applies only to the elderly, excludes all but a small fraction of the homeless.

The Medicaid programme (Title XIX of the Social Security Act) is a means-tested health care benefit for the indigent which is funded jointly by the federal and state governments and administered at the state level. Although the federal government requires the states to provide Medicaid health benefits for certain groups, such as the blind or disabled or some single parents with dependent children, the over-

50 Medicaid programmes are free to define requirements for eligibility. As a result, there are great differences in coverage as one compares one state to another. Across the country, less than 40 per cent of poor people receive any Medicaid benefits.

As a result of the health care insurance problems in the country, at least 35,000,000 Americans under age 65 have no public or private insurance coverage during at least part of each year. Further complicating these problems is the increasing pressure being brought to bear on hospitals to decrease their commitment to providing care for people who cannot pay. This pressure arises from the fact that the cost of medical care has doubled in the past decade, increasing cost-control strategies are being demanded by employers and the federal government, thereby decreasing hospital profits, and, finally, the size of the uninsured population, many of whom are homeless, has increased by at least 1,000,000 per year since 1980.

Traditionally, many communities have attempted to fill the gaps in provision of health care for the poor by the establishment of public hospitals in major urban areas. These hospitals, and their associated clinics, have served as a provider-of-last-resort for many medically indigent and homeless individuals for decades. However, due to the declining federal support for local government services, the increasing demand for health services and the competitive nature of health care in the United States, many local government health departments have closed their hospitals because of the huge financial drain which they represent. As a result, less than 50 per cent of the major urban areas in the United States now have a public hospital. These closures have had a disproportionate impact on the homeless who have often relied on urban public hospital emergency rooms as their only source of care. Private hospitals, attempting to minimize their financial losses from care of medically indigent and homeless people, have engaged in the practice of dumping uninsured patients on local public hospitals (Ansell and Schiff 1987). Without the availability of a public hospital, the homeless may be sent back out on the street from the emergency room rather than being admitted to the hospital where their charges cannot be recovered by the hospital.

A final avenue of health care for homeless individuals and the medically indigent is the system co-ordinated by the Department of Veterans' Affairs (VA). Veterans of military service are eligible for various health care benefits through the system of 172 hospitals and clinics nationwide co-ordinated by the Department of Veterans' Affairs. The services are free of charge and, in many instances, comprehensive. In many aspects, the VA health care system is the closest approximation to a national health programme for a defined segment of the American population. As up to one-third of the homeless in the United States are veterans, the VA system is a resource in many communities for medically indigent homeless veterans in need of health care.

Homelessness magnifies the problems of health care financing and delivery in the United States. The vast majority of the homeless, whether single or in families, do not receive public cash assistance of Medicaid benefits and face both financial and physical barriers to access to health care. Although continuous comprehensive primary care, a cornerstone of the National Health Service, remains beyond the reach of many in the United States, the homeless are even less likely to receive such care and yet are in the greatest need. Complicating these issues is the fact that many homeless people are sceptical, or afraid, of institutions, including those for health care. For these reasons, special programmes have been developed to overcome these obstacles.

## HISTORICAL DEVELOPMENTS

Historically, three issues underpin the development of special health care programmes for the homeless. First, the organization of health care in the United States, with institutional policies requiring payment for services, excludes the homeless for financial reasons. Second, the special needs of the homeless population, including geographic isolation and transportation barriers, are not well accommodated by the model of the hospital-based clinic for the indigent. Lastly, attitudes of health care professionals have frequently labelled the homeless as an undesirable group of patients, further estranging this high-risk and medically needy population from traditional services.

In 1969, the St Vincent's Hospital and Medical Centre in New York City pioneered the concept of health care teams which were based on the principle of outreach contact with an individual who would otherwise be unserved. At its inception, this programme focused on homeless individuals living in large, low-income SRO hotels in the Skid Row area of New York City. The outreach teams, comprised of physicians, nurses, social workers, health professional students and other service providers, brought their services to the hotels where they conducted clinics, often in marginal accommodation with few of the amenities of traditional medical practice. These clinics were an attempt to treat problems early in their course on-site and, therefore, to decrease the frequency of acute crises and fragmented and episodic care and to encourage independent use of the more traditional health care system while preserving dignity and humanity. These outreach workers, who often visited the homeless in their temporary quarters, were backed up by the shelter- or hotel-based health station and hospital-based clinics at St Vincent's Hospital. Over the past two decades, this programme has continued to serve as a model for other programmes and now involves over twenty-five sites. The experience of the St Vincent's Programme served as a basis for the first comprehensive text on health care for the homeless in the United States (Brickner *et al.* 1985).

The St Vincent's Programme exemplifies the role that a major affiliated health care centre, with a mission to serve the poor, can play in a local community to expand health care resources for the homeless. Unfortunately, few other communities in the United States enjoy this level of commitment from their local hospitals. Throughout many urban areas in the country, the homeless continue to experience episodic assessment and treatment obtained in the crisis-orientated settings of urban emergency rooms. In most locales, programmes to serve the homeless have been initiated by the non-profit, or voluntary, sector. During the 1970s and expanding in the 1980s as an outgrowth of the community health clinic concept, non-profit programmes developed to fill the gaps in health care delivery for the poor and the homeless. Most of these programmes were initiated by churches or other religious groups or formed by the commitment of one or two individuals. Many of these non-profit programmes operate in the evening hours because of their dependence on volunteer health care professionals to provide services.

The benefits of such non-profit programmes include the on-site services which are provided where the homeless congregate, either emergency shelters, SRO hotels or streets and parks in the case of mobile van units. A major function of these non-profit programmes is to serve as a mechanism for advocacy for the homeless, helping them to gain access to more traditional services when health problems exceed what can be provided by these small groups (Reuler *et al.* 1986). As outlined by the Institute of Medicine Report, however, these non-profit initiatives, though well intentioned, suffer from the problems of limited hours, reliance on volunteers and limited access to medications and ancillary services. Additionally, most of the programmes suffer from great instability in their bases and lack the ability to provide any form of systematic preventive care beyond treatment of acute problems. More recently, the viability of such programmes has also been threatened by the potential withdrawal of malpractice insurance coverage by insurance carriers. Staff burn-out in such frontline programmes is a common occurrence.

As the 1980s began, cutbacks in federal government support of local communities and the increasing size of the homeless population began to place great strains on the fragile balance supported by these voluntary sector programmes. The increasing demands on the resources of county (local government) health departments and the early public health implications of human immunodeficiency virus (HIV) infection limited public sector development of health programmes for the homeless. As well, the growing homeless population in core urban areas led to conflicts between programmes developing community multi-service centres for the homeless and local business interests which often viewed the homeless as deterrents to successful business enterprise. These increasing problems led to the search, both nationally and locally, for creative solutions to the myriad problems, including health care, facing the homeless.

## THE JOHNSON-PEW PROGRAMME

1983 dawned with tremendous attention being focused on the plight of the homeless. Not only had the U.S. Conference of Mayors' report and Congressional hearings on homelessness received great press coverage over the holiday season, but also the havoc wrought by the policies of the new federal administration underscored the inability of existing agencies to serve the needs of the homeless. The Robert Wood Johnson Foundation, one of the nation's largest private philanthropies which devotes its resources to solutions to the health care problems in the U.S., identified health care for the homeless as a national priority requiring development of innovative solutions. In conjunction with the Pew Charitable Trusts, one of the U.S.'s largest general funds, and co-sponsored by the U.S. Conference of Mayors, the Robert Wood Johnson Foundation announced, in December 1983, a Health Care for the Homeless Competitive Grant Programme open to the fifty-one largest cities in the United States. The development of the grant programme was predicated on the conclusions that health care for the homeless was sorely needed and largely unavailable; that, without good health, homeless people cannot resolve their other basic problems; and that health care programmes for the homeless could be effective when conducted in appropriate settings and combined with other services and benefits. In order to overcome problems which had plagued health care for the homeless programmes in other settings, the Foundation initiative mandated that applicant cities meet the following basic criteria: first, that an overall strategy for delivery of health and social services be developed, which included specific on-site service delivery located in shelters or other locations where homeless congregated and that the efforts be co-ordinated by a core service team of physicians and nurses with social workers and other service providers. Second, applicants must demonstrate that there is a city-wide coalition responsible for the design and implementation of the programme. Third, welfare and housing agencies, in addition to health care providers, must be involved in programme activities. Lastly, specific plans were to be outlined for continuing support of the programme when grant funding terminated at the end of four years (Brickner *et al.* 1990).

One year after announcing the request for proposals, grants were awarded to nineteen cities, each receiving $1.4 million for the duration of the programme. A notable aspect of the Johnson-Pew initiative was that it forced local governments to form effective coalitions to deal with co-ordination of health care and other services for the homeless. Few cities had such coalitions in place prior to the announcement of request for proposals. Also, the foundations committed additional funding to support a research arm of this project and contracted with the Social and Demography Research Institute of the University of Massachusetts to complete this analysis.

The fundamental principle of most of the project programmes was that of case management, a mechanism for facilitating access and movement of an individual through fragmented service systems. The Johnson-Pew initiative raised many questions about the need to develop separate health care systems for the homeless, similar to discussions within the National Health Service about health care programmes relying upon salaried general practitioners. Unifying themes among the nineteen programmes included a holistic approach using the outreach concept delivered by empathetic staff and an interdisciplinary team. A broad range of health and social services was provided in most programmes along with major attempts at strengthening continuity through case management principles.

Despite similar themes, the projects of the nineteen cities reflected the individual needs of each locale. This concept of local solutions and outreach to the community is similar to that envisioned by the Department of Health (DoH) in the development of the two health care for single homeless schemes in London. Several aspects of the programmes differed significantly from one city to another. First, the form of governance of these programmes varied, including the establishment of a separate non-profit board to oversee the programme, the incorporation of the programme under existing health care or social service agencies or the assignment of one of the local charities, such as a community foundation, to oversee and administer the programme. Similarly, the manner of administration ranged between direct provision of services by staff employed by the programme to the contracting out of service delivery to separate health and social service agencies existent in the local area. The structure and management dynamics of many of these programmes, particularly during the early period of implementation, mirrored many of the problems encountered in the DHSS demonstration projects in London (Williams and Allen 1989). These included blurred lines of accountability or clearly defined lines of responsibility within multidisciplinary teams. Finally, the methods of operation varied between having centralized clinics located at shelters and hotels to mobile teams working out of vans visiting streets and parks to engage the homeless in participation in the programme.

During the four years of the nineteen demonstration projects, the problems of the homeless in the United States continued to grow. In certain urban areas, the HIV problem within the homeless community became a paramount concern of health delivery agencies. Notwithstanding the growing size of the homeless population and competing demands for limited funding options, the majority of the coalition programmes were able to capture funding to preserve most of the programmes beyond the four years of Johnson-Pew support. Despite initial issues with programme governance at the local levels, a clear success of this initiative has been the forging of coalitions for the homeless in many cities which previously had suffered from poor communication among agencies and between agencies and local government. This coalition building, forged by the Johnson-Pew programmes, will serve as a template for facing the continuing challenges for adequate health care for the homeless in the 1990s.

## HEALTH PROBLEMS OF THE HOMELESS

Because of their vulnerability and barriers to access to health services, the homeless shoulder the highest burden of untreated illness in the United States. The medical problems of the homeless are often common afflictions magnified by chaotic living conditions (Brickner *et al.* 1986). Until recently, most literature on health problems in the homeless was comprised primarily of anecdotal experience and commentary. However, more recent longitudinal studies of the homeless and the information from the Johnson-Pew programmes have underscored previous observations of the poor health of the homeless (Gelberg and Linn 1989; Wright and Weber 1987).

In the Social and Demographic Research Institute analysis of sixteen Johnson-Pew sites through the first two years of the programme, 63,000 clients were evaluated out of 100,000 patients seen during that period. Two-thirds of the visits were for acute problems, and one-third for chronic conditions, similar to findings of the National Ambulatory Medical Care Survey conducted in 1979 and to which the Johnson-Pew analysis was compared. Of the acute medical problems, upper respiratory infections accounted for one-third, trauma for one-quarter and skin conditions for 14 per cent. Alcohol abuse was the number one health problem, seen in 38 per cent of the population total, with 47 per cent of men and 16 per cent of women being alcohol abusers. Chronic mental illness was seen in one-third of patients. Women were twice as likely as men to have chronic mental illness, whereas men were three times more likely than women to have chronic alcohol abuse. Thirteen per cent of the population had a history of drug abuse other than alcohol. Forty-one per cent of the patients seen in the Johnson-Pew programmes suffered from chronic medical problems, including hypertension, gastro-intestinal disorders, peripheral vascular disease and dental disease, compared to 25 per cent of those domiciled adults seen in office practice during the National Ambulatory Medical Care Survey.

Additional analysis of the Health Care for the Homeless projects' experience compared to that of the National Ambulatory Medical Care Survey showed that the homeless were six times as likely to have a neurological disorder, five times as likely to have hepatitis, four times as likely to have respiratory or nutritional disorders and two to three times as likely to have skin problems or suffer from trauma. Of the eighty-seven deaths analysed, homicide or trauma accounted for the majority, and the death rate among this sample of the homeless was three to four times that of the general population, with an average age of death 22 years younger than that in the general population. Also, the degree of functional limitation has been shown to be greater in the homeless compared to domiciled poor (Gelberg *et al.* 1990).

Examination of causes of hospitalization of homeless individuals has shown that the homeless suffer from disorders of the extremities fifteen times the rate of the national population and that cellulitis is one of the most common problems leading to hospitalization of the homeless (Morris and Crystal 1989). Additionally, the homeless, when compared to poor people who are housed, are more likely to be hospitalized for mental illness, substance abuse or delirium tremens.

Tuberculosis is another problem afflicting the homeless, a result of crowded living conditions, inadequate nutrition and the effect of chronic stress on the immune system. Mycobacterium tuberculosis infection in the homeless is twenty-five to fifty times that of urban adults who are domiciled and one hundred times that of all U.S. adults. Additionally, 8 per cent of the homeless in some studies have been shown to have active pulmonary tuberculosis. Adequate treatment of this latter group is particularly complicated given the frequently encountered combination of chronic mental illness, the nomadic lifestyle of many homeless people and institutional barriers to health care assessment and follow-up (Schieffelbein and Snider 1988). The problem of tuberculosis is particularly relevant to the homeless with HIV infection. Although the true prevalence of HIV infection in the homeless is not known, in New York City, 62 per cent of a group of 169 high-risk homeless individuals were found to be HIV positive (Torres *et al.* 1990). In large urban areas like Los Angeles and New York City, the numbers of HIV-infected individuals among the homeless will likely increase as high-risk groups and minorities are disproportionately represented.

Homeless children represent a special subset of the homeless population who are particularly vulnerable (Alperstein and Arnstein 1988). Homeless children are four times more likely to be in fair or poor health compared to housed children, are twice as likely to be unimmunized and are much less likely to have had tuberculin skin testing or regular dental care. In addition to the physical sequelae of homelessness, increasing attention has been focused on the psychological impact of homelessness on children (Lewis and Meyers 1989). The stress of homelessness increases the risk of substance abuse and child abuse within the family, causing depression, behavioural changes, distrust of adults and poor school performance. The frequency of acute and chronic medical problems and the prevalence of nutritional deficiencies in homeless children further magnify the psychological scars to homelessness for this group (Miller and Lin 1988).

Homeless street youth also represent a high-risk group (Council on Scientific Affairs, AMA 1989). These teenagers have often escaped physical, sexual and emotional abuse at home prior to entering street life and often engage in high-risk behaviour such as prostitution and intravenous substance abuse. Though many of the problems encountered in street youth are common acute problems of that age group in general, engaging this alienated population in traditional health services has posed a great challenge. This has been particularly the case with delivery of prenatal care to pregnant homeless teens, all of whom represent very high-risk pregnancies.

## VA HOMELESS MENTALLY ILL PROGRAMME

The Johnson-Pew programme represented a private initiative with a national scope. At the time that initial experience with these nineteen projects was being examined, a federal government programme to aid the homeless was launched on a national scale. Public Law 100-6 established the Department of Veterans' Affairs' Homeless Chronically Mentally Ill Programme and committed $5 million to support the endeavour. This represented the largest integrated treatment initiative for the homeless mentally ill in the country.

In the spring of 1987, projects under this sponsorship were implemented at forty-three medical centres across the U.S. Recognizing the extreme disaffiliation that comes with being homeless and chronically mentally ill and a veteran of the Vietnam campaign, this national programme was anchored in the concept of a commonly orientated health care delivery system. As a result, effective linkage between a government hospital and community-based health and social services was established. The VA Programme was comprised of six components: aggressive outreach to make contact with the chronically mentally ill; intake assessments, including eligibility and needs; specialized psychiatric and medical evaluation; referral to VA and non-VA psychiatric and medical treatment facilities; residential treatment, contracted out to non-VA centres, for up to one year; and case management and advocacy.

Each programme included VA clinicians and administrative support personnel. During the first two years, 19,697 homeless veterans were assessed (Rosenheck *et al.* 1989). The average age was 42.6 years, and 51 per cent served during the Vietnam campaign. As with the homeless in general, alcohol abuse was a major problem, seen in 44 per cent of those evaluated. One-third had been hospitalized for psychiatric illness other than substance abuse and one-tenth met diagnostic criteria for post-traumatic stress disorder. The prevalence of acute and chronic medical conditions was even greater than in the general population, a finding corroborated by other recent data about homelessness (Gelberg *et al.* 1988; Breakey *et al.* 1989). Over 6 per cent of patients were judged to require acute hospitalization at the time of intake assessment.

The VA's programme demonstrated several things. First, the number of veterans seen at a locale correlates with the intensity and scope of outreach. This point reiterated the fact that it is possible to engage the homeless in a professional system of health care which uses a community-based model. Second, outreach is very staff-intensive and, with this population, very stressful for staff. Special staffing patterns and support are required to assure success and continuity. Third, residential treatment of this highly vulnerable mentally ill population led to improvement in over one-half of patients. Finally, most programme sites found that the availability of community residential treatment facilities was grossly inadequate, mirroring the nationwide frustration of non-profit homeless care programmes attempting to place patients with mental illness or substance abuse into treatment. This latter problem was eased by the subsequent establishment of twenty-six domiciliary units in the VA system under Public Law 100–71, the Domiciliary Care for Homeless Veterans programme.

## THE McKINNEY ACT

In response to the increasing problem of homelessness across the country and the leadership provided by private initiatives, such as the Johnson-Pew model, the U.S. Congress, in July 1987, passed the first major legislation to respond to the special needs of the homeless. Called the Stewart B. McKinney Homeless Assistance Act (Public Law 100–77), this bill established an Interagency Council on the Homeless with a mandate to: review all federal activities and programmes to assist homeless individuals; reduce duplication among programmes and activities by federal agencies; monitor evaluations and recommend improvements in programmes and activities conducted by federal agencies, state and local governments and private voluntary agencies; provide professional and technical assistance to states, local government and public and private non-profit organizations; collect and disseminate information; and report annually to Congress on the extent and nature of homelessness.

In addition to housing and educational components, Title VI of the McKinney Act is devoted to primary health services and community mental health services for the homeless. Availability of McKinney funds became one mechanism for many of the Johnson-Pew programmes to continue service delivery at the end of their four-year grant cycle. In fiscal year 1991, $819 million was allocated by the Congress to support all McKinney Act initiatives around the country. However, this level of funding is only a fraction of that necessary to support ongoing homeless programmes in local communities, and the stability of the funding is uncertain, as these funds must compete with many other programmes funded by the federal government in a time of an enlarging federal deficit and decreasing federal support for many local government programmes. The effectiveness of the Interagency Council in streamlining the grant review process and lessening the burden of paperwork on overstretched, frontline service delivery staff is awaiting evaluation.

## FUTURE DIRECTIONS

Although the absence of a nationalized health programme represents a significant difference between the United States and Great Britain, health care for the homeless in both countries shares similar features. Inadequate housing remains the root problem for many of the health-related consequences of homelessness, and the health care system, in and of itself, cannot rectify this ill. Also, in both countries, it has been shown that outreach to this vulnerable population is essential to assure adequate access to health services.

The primary care model, which assures access, comprehensiveness, co-ordination and integration of services and continuity, is particularly important for the homeless, as the specialist-orientated, institutionally-based services characteristic of U.S. health care pose great barriers for this group. However, the health care for the homeless projects around the country which have evolved over the past two decades have focused on the model of non-profit agencies providing stop-gap emergency services. What is needed now is a shift to more government involvement and support, with a focus towards long-term solutions.

One challenge for the future is to develop a more comprehensive strategy encompassing the heterogeneity of the homeless population. The sub-groups of the homeless differ greatly *vis-à-vis* sociodemographic characteristics, health perception and prior experiences. Effectively meeting the needs of these disparate units will require development of appropriate programmes and interventions. The emergency shelter/SRO hotel-based clinic model orientated to the single adult homeless male may not be relevant for the majority of homeless people in the U.S. today. This is particularly true for the enlarging population of rural homeless.

The chronically mentally ill represent a poignant failure of health services delivery, and homelessness is just one symptom of the problems facing this group. The American Psychiatric Association's call for a comprehensive and integrated system of care for the chronically mentally ill homeless, with designated responsibility, accountability and adequate fiscal resources, is yet to be realized (Lamb and Talbott 1986). The experiences of general health care programmes for the homeless continue to highlight the fragility of the chronically mentally ill and the difficulty in providing any semblance of care for them in the construct of a loose network of services rather than a true system of care.

Reflecting on the U.S. experience over the past decade, progress has been made in improving health care to the homeless population. Innovative programmes have demonstrated that effective partnerships can be forged among diverse agencies and that local advocacy and outreach can embrace a generally disenfranchised group. However, short-term solutions will not resolve the long-term problems resulting from inadequate housing and absence of a universal health care system for the population. The increasing size of the homeless population, the competitive nature of the for-profit health industry and the complexion of administration and congressional budget priorities in recent years place any gains that have been made in great jeopardy. Voluntary agencies cannot shoulder the societal burden of health care for the homeless without reliable and substantial support from government. This will be the major challenge for the coming years.

## REFERENCES

Alperstein, G. and Arnstein, E. (1988) 'Homeless children – a challenge for pediatricians', *The Pediatric Clinics of North America* 35: 1413-25.

Ansell, D. A. and Schiff, R. L. (1987) 'Patient dumping – status, implications and policy recommendations', *Journal of the American Medical Association* 257: 1500-2.

Bachrach, L. L. (1987) 'Homeless women: a context for health planning', *The Milbank Quarterly* 65: 371-97.

Bassuk, E. L. and Rosenberg, L. (1988) 'Why does family homelessness occur? A case-control study', *American Journal of Public Health* 78: 783-8.

Breakey, W. R., Fischer, P. J., Kramer, M., Nestadt, G., Romanoski, A. J., Ross, A., Royall, R M. and Stine, O C. (1989) 'Health and mental health problems of homeless men and women in Baltimore', *Journal of the American Medical Association* 262: 1352-7.

Brickner, P. W., Scanlan, B. C., Conanan, B., Elvy, A., MacAdam, J., Scharer, L. K. and Vicic, W. J. (1986) 'Homeless persons and health care', *Annals of Internal Medicine* 104: 405-9.

Brickner, P. W., Scharer, L. K., Conanan, B., Elvy, A. and Savarese, M. (eds) (1985) *Health Care of Homeless People*, New York: Springer.

Brickner, P. W., Scharer, L. K., Conanan, B. A., Savarese, M. and Scanlan, B. C. (eds) (1990) *Under the Safety Net – The Health and Social Welfare of the Homeless in the United States*, New York: Norton.

Council on Scientific Affairs, American Medical Association (1989) 'Health care needs of homeless and runaway youths', *Journal of the American Medical Association* 262: 1358–61.

Fein, R. (1986) *Medical Costs – The Search for a Health Insurance Policy*, Cambridge, MA: Harvard University Press.

Gelberg, L. and Linn, L. S. (1989) 'Assessing the physical health of homeless adults', *Journal of the American Medical Association* 262:1973–9.

Gelberg, L., Linn, L. S., and Leake, B. D. (1988) 'Mental health, alcohol and drug use, and criminal history among homeless adults', *American Journal of Psychiatry* 145: 191–6.

Gelberg, L., Linn, L. S., Usatine, R. P. and Smith, M. H. (1990) 'Health, homelessness, and poverty – a study of clinic users', *Archives of Internal Medicine* 150: 2325–30.

Institute of Medicine (1988) *Homelessness, Health, and Human Needs*, Washington, DC: National Academy Press.

Lamb, H. R. (ed.) (1984) *The Homeless Mentally Ill*, Washington, DC: American Psychiatric Association.

Lamb, H. R. and Talbott, J. A. (1986) 'The homeless mentally ill – the perspective of the American Psychiatric Association', *Journal of the American Medical Association* 256: 498–501.

Lewis, M. R. and Meyers, A. F. (1989) 'The growth and development status of homeless children entering shelters in Boston', *Public Health Reports* 104: 247–50.

Linn, L. S. and Gelberg, L. (1989) 'Priority of basic needs among homeless adults', *Social Psychiatry and Psychiatric Epidemiology* 24: 23–9.

Linn, L. S., Gelberg, L. and Leake, B. (1990) 'Substance abuse and mental health status of homeless and domiciled low-income users of a medical clinic', *Hospital and Community Psychiatry* 41: 306–10.

Miller, D. S. and Lin, E. H. B. (1988) 'Children in sheltered homeless families: reported health status and use of health services', *Pediatrics* 81: 668–73.

Morris, W. and Crystal, S. (1989) 'Diagnostic patterns in hospital use by an urban homeless population', *Western Journal of Medicine* 151: 472–6.

Reuler, J. B., Bax, M. J. and Sampson, J. H. (1986) 'Physician house call services for medically needy, inner-city residents', *American Journal of Public Health* 76: 1131–4.

Robertson, M. J. and Cousineau, M. R. (1986) 'Health status and access to health services among the urban homeless', *American Journal of Public Health* 76: 561–3.

Rosenheck, R., Leda, C., Gallup, P., Astrachan, B., Milstein, R., Leaf, P., Thompson, D. and Errera, P. (1989) 'Initial assessment data from a 43-site programme for chronic mentally ill veterans', *Hospital and Community Psychiatry* 40: 937–42.

Schieffelbein, C. W. and Snider, D. E. (1988) 'Tuberculosis control among homeless populations', *Archives of Internal Medicine* 148: 1843–6.

Torres, R. A., Mani, S., Altholz, J. and Brickner, P. W. (1990) 'Human immunodeficiency virus infection among homeless men in New York City shelter – association with mycobacterium tuberculosis infection', *Archives of Internal Medicine* 150: 2030–6.

Weinreb, L. F. and Bassuk, E. L. (1990) 'Health care of homeless families – a growing challenge for family medicine', *The Journal of Family Practice* 31: 74–80.

Williams, S. and Allen, I. (1989) *Health Care for Single Homeless People*, London: Policy Studies Institute.

Wood, D., Valdez, B., Hayashi, T. and Shen, A. (1990) 'Homeless and housed families in Los Angeles: a study comparing demographic, economic and family function characteristics', *American Journal of Public Health* 80: 1049–52.

Wright, J. D. (1989) *Address Unknown – The Homeless in America*, New York: Aldine de Gruyter.

Wright, J. D. and Weber, E. (1987) *Homelessness and Health*, Washington, DC: McGraw-Hill.

# Conclusion

*John Collins*

Inadequate housing provision, including, most importantly, the lack of *affordable* accommodation available for rent in both urban and rural areas, remains the fundamental cause of all homelessness. This is also the underlying cause of many of the adverse consequences upon the health of single homeless people. These truths, we have seen, are found to apply equally both here and in the USA. It is also evident that the 'shape' and scale of the 'problem' of homelessness are largely a consequence of social policy in housing, social welfare, benefit and health care systems.

In the UK we have many homeless families housed in unsatisfactory temporary accommodation by local authorities unable to provide them with permanent secure and satisfactory homes because of inadequate housing 'stock' in the public sector. These families have many housing-related health problems and because of their concentration and geographical isolation in 'hotel ghettos' often also have problems accessing health care. Indeed, in the USA 50 per cent of such families would be totally dependent on charitable health care provision, whereas in the UK statutory responsibility for provision of housing to families with children facilitates their integration into local mainstream health care services. This work has not attempted to explore the specific problems facing homeless families seeking health care, but it is precisely because of the fact that social policy makes no statutory provision to meet the housing needs of adults under 65 (unless they can be deemed 'vulnerable and in priority need') that the problems of access to health care for single homeless people are qualitatively different from those confronting homeless families though, obviously, there are themes common to both. The prevailing social 'culture' in the UK demands that single people should be wholly independent and, as adults, self-supporting. Our welfare benefits system is evidence of this collective expectation and several authors here have shown how the recent changes in benefit arrangements for young people have conspired to effect an increase in the numbers of young single homeless people sleeping rough in urban areas and the health-related consequences of this lifestyle. Even if these policies were quickly reversed, the long-term effects on the current young homeless will take years to settle and there will undoubtedly be a group of people permanently socially 'disabled' by their experiences whose health will suffer in consequence. We have shown how social antagonism to single homeless people leads to a profound loss of self-esteem and stigmatization. The behavioural consequences of this loss of self-worth, e.g. withdrawal, street drinking, drug abuse, combined with the effects of poverty, illiteracy and lifestyle on personal presentation, frequently conspire to reinforce social justification in blaming the victim. The existence of this 'vicious circle of social expectation' may then be used to excuse the failure of health and social services to respond: response is 'pointless', the victims 'unhelpable' and the problem containable only by further marginalization, conveniently facilitated by the poor self-advocacy of single homeless people themselves, their lack of health awareness and isolation.

It is in this complex milieu of social forces that primary care providers of all disciplines operate. Health care is not the principal determinant of health but an awareness of the significant health care needs of single homeless people has given rise to a range of responses by various agents. We have seen how barriers to access arise from structural, administrative and attitudinal problems within the NHS itself and also how personal and perceptual factors conspire to prevent single homeless people from seeking health care services.

Historically, awareness of these difficulties and pressure for improvement in health care provision began in the philanthropic tradition and became the responsibility of the voluntary sector. Ad hoc and varied responses developed to meet the needs of single homeless people, initially based on the 'workhouse' model involving imposition of provision built on assumptions of need (in both housing and health care). Later, with the development of the NHS and post-war social policy, gradual changes in our perceptions of 'the problem' have occurred. These changes, initially largely forced by pioneering enthusiasts in the field and continued by the development of campaigning, have gradually shifted the emphasis away from marginal solutions, special clinics, hostels and services, to the recognition that mainstream services should make flexible and imaginative local responses to need based on outreach, advocacy and collaborative working methods. Is this right? Are we just setting a trend here? Might single homeless people not be better served by specialist services provided for them alone? These are important questions with no self-evident answers and it is clear that philosophical re-orientation alone does not produce material change. Our own feeling, based on our experience at HHELP working in the East End of London, is that specialist services are part of the dynamic process of change and take their place on a continuum of development. They are valid as a statutory response to the pragmatic need to provide health care service to unregistered single homeless people, but they are largely still dependent on 'enthusiasts' for their existence and rely on 'project' or other short-term funding arrangements. The usefulness of statutory specialist services is that they can, if correctly managed, perform a dual role of providing services and influencing service providers by their day to day work, referrals, etc., by providing a training/education resource and a research base within the statutory sector. For health care professionals the aim of integration is a long-term one and, as we have said, dependent on changes within housing and social policy, but it is the only sensible aim, one which would reinforce self-advocacy and health awareness among single homeless people and foster their empowerment.

This is not to say that specialist teams are either easy to manage or always successful or, necessarily, a model response for all areas. The HHELP team, having grown from a project, has been successful in East London largely because of the pre-existing voluntary sector network and the goodwill of local statutory providers. Elsewhere more rapid progress to integration into mainstream NHS services may be achievable. We have always felt that in primary care local responses to local needs are likely to be most appropriate and successful and reference to 'models' in this context displays a lack of empathy for the problems of access to care.

## THE FUTURE

A common theme throughout this book is that the access to, and quality of, health care provision for single homeless people would be enhanced by the development of flexible, integrated, multidisciplinary primary care services with outreach and advocacy functions built in.

The 1991 NHS reforms, in separating purchaser and provider functions, present an opportunity for the development of such an approach, at the purchaser level, if purchasers can be persuaded to prioritize services for single homeless people.

Already some FHSAs and purchasing DHA units are moving

towards an integrated approach and this has much potential to improve matters given the necessary resources. It is arguable too that social care provision should be included under this umbrella with the reintegration of local authority social and home care services into the NHS management structure (having been removed in the 1974 NHS reorganization), though there are no plans for this at present. Joint planning arrangements involving district health authorities/FHSAs and local authorities will remain and are central to the forthcoming (1992) inception of the community care arrangements for the development of community services for the mentally ill, elderly, disabled and children. The major concern of those involved in improving care provision to single homeless people is that, if purchasing resources are inadequate and/or completely decentralized to fund-holding general practitioners, prioritizing the development of integrative services for this (and other) disadvantaged groups will become even more difficult than at present. Only effective self-advocacy would protect against this and single homeless people are, both as individuals and as a group, especially unlikely to exhibit effective self-advocacy skills.

The NHS *Patient's Charter* 1991 lists nine standards of service which the NHS aims to provide. One of these is that 'arrangements should ensure everyone, including people with special needs, can use the services available'. Effective representation of the needs of homeless people within service management structures is essential if this aim is to be achieved with respect to the single homeless community.

Community care planning and the NHS reforms along with the 1990 new contract for NHS general practitioners will all have significant effects on health care provision for single homeless people. Some of those effects are as yet unpredictable.

The separation of purchaser and provider functions provides an opportunity for services in the community to become more flexible and integrated. If the resources are made available to enhance a co-ordinated multidisciplinary approach to health care for single homeless people then there is every prospect of improving access and morbidity. Purchasers' other priorities are a worry since the effective representation of the needs of homeless people to purchasers is still likely to depend on enthusiasts and concerned third parties in the voluntary sector. Such representation is likely to be marginalized in favour of spending in other 'high profile' areas of health care.

In contrast, the general practitioner contract of 1990 – which was forced on general practitioners by the then Secretary of State for Health – has had a detrimental effect on access to GP services for homeless people generally. This seems to have come about for a variety of complex reasons, many of which where foreseen by workers in the field:

1 The contract has made GPs generally much busier as have the 1991 reforms and therefore reluctant to take on any 'extra' work.

2 Although the proportion of a GP's income derived from his/her patient list has increased, which, in theory, should make them keener to accept new and additional patients, this effect has, in inner-city areas, been outweighed by other conflicting aspects of the contract.

3 Deprivation payments were introduced to offset some of the financial penalties of general practice in inner cities compared to suburban and rural areas. Patients resident in certain electoral wards, deemed high and medium deprivation areas by use of the Jarman score, earn a supplementary fee for the GP. NFA patients are, unfortunately, not included since they do not have a post code. This acts as a direct disincentive to permanent registration.

4 Target payments. GPs now receive 'bonus' payments if they achieve a fixed percentage of cervical smear tests on eligible (16–64 years) women on their practice lists. Women who are mobile, non-compliant or addressless are perceived to disadvantage the doctor's chances of achieving his/her target. This acts as a disincentive to register NFA/homeless women.

5 GP budget holding. Only a relatively small number of urban practices (and therefore patients) are affected by this change to date. The doctors involved manage their own budget, allocated in advance, and purchase all non-emergency care for their patients (up to an arbitrary cost limit in each case of £5,000). This has not proved a popular arrangement with inner-city GPs anywhere in the country and clearly, if the arrangement became widespread, unregistered patients might find it very hard to access non-emergency care and, as we have seen, about three-quarters of street dwellers are unregistered with a GP at any one time.

The unpredictability of the outcome of these various legislative and practical changes makes service provision in the NHS presently even more difficult than hitherto and this is especially true in providing primary care to homeless people. The mobility of some groups of homeless people makes them very vulnerable to arguments about 'catchment areas' when approaching purchasing authorities for the provision of non-urgent care. Budget limitations for extra contractual referrals – that is, referrals to providers with whom the purchaser has no existing contract, for instance to a specialist alcohol or drug treatment facility some distance away from the locality – are already causing constraints on GP referral freedoms in some areas. Furthermore, in some areas non-medical health care professionals cannot now refer independently without the 'sponsorship' of the patient's GP – difficult if the patient is unregistered and does not themselves see registration as a priority for whatever reason.

## THE WAY AHEAD

In order to help homeless single people in a way that enables and empowers them, increasingly, to further help themselves should, logically, be based on a care planning approach. This approach (SSI 1990) which has developed from the American work of Stein and Test (1980) involves multidisciplinary contributions co-ordinated for an individual by a named and accessible key worker. This key worker may be from any professional, or possibly also lay, background but needs a relationship with the client/patient which is capable of fostering that client's on-going personal growth and development.

With regard to single homeless people we feel that community care planning teams should, as necessary, involve all relevant statutory health professionals. This should result in more and more appropriate interventions made in a way which is much more likely to coincide with the client's perception of their own needs and avoid the trap of providing 'programmed care' which is, or may become, conditional on meeting criteria which the client cannot fulfil.

In order for such a personalized system of health and social care to work, then obviously much more flexibility is required within the housing, welfare, benefit and educational structures to encompass people's diverse needs. This may require a greater input of public money, but more importantly requires the development of structures and roles which allow financial, medical, housing and social resources to be used imaginatively for the benefit of individuals. Housing and resettlement workers, voluntary sector personnel, social care staff and representatives with educational and training skills, as well as health care professionals need to be involved, flexibly, in the care planning approach.

Any individual single homeless person may have one or, more likely, a complex range of personal, social, psychological and medical problems. No single professional worker, working in isolation, is likely to be able to make more than a perfunctory intervention in these circumstances. The single homeless client will sometimes have very different perceptions, beliefs and frames of reference from those of the health worker. Confusion and misunderstanding result. Care and development are impeded.

Care planning offers an opportunity for advocates, with expert help, to prioritize a person's range of problems and for a co-ordinated planned approach to them to be developed rather than, as hitherto, the needs of individuals being put second to those of the provider.

We can finish as we began! Single homeless people need housing. They are not 'of a type' and so a range of housing provision needs to be available and accessible to them. Not until such facilities exist will their social, psychological and physical needs begin to be met. Only when these needs are met will their health improve.

## REFERENCES

Department of Health (1991a) *The Patient's Charter*, London: HMSO.
Department of Health (1991b) *The NHS Reforms*, London: HMSO.
Social Services Inspectorate (1990) *Community Care in the Next Decade and Beyond*, London: DOH, SSI.
Stein, L. and Test, M.A. (1980) 'Alternatives to mental hospital treatment', *Archives of General Psychiatry* 37: 392–7.

# Name index

# Subject index